Santería Healing

Contemporary Cuba

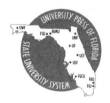

Florida A&M University, Tallahassee
Florida Atlantic University, Boca Raton
Florida Gulf Coast University, Ft. Myers
Florida International University, Miami
Florida State University, Tallahassee
University of Central Florida, Orlando
University of Florida, Gainesville
University of North Florida, Jacksonville
University of South Florida, Tampa
University of West Florida, Pensacola

Contemporary Cuba
Edited by John M. Kirk

Santería Healing

A Journey into the Afro-Cuban World
of Divinities, Spirits, and Sorcery

Johan Wedel

University Press of Florida
Gainesville · Tallahassee · Tampa · Boca Raton
Pensacola · Orlando · Miami · Jacksonville · Ft. Myers

This book is an informational guide and not intended for
medicating or curing ailments of any kind. Its purpose is only
illustrative. Neither the author nor the publisher recommends
using any of the remedies or techniques discussed in the book.

09 08 07 06 05 04   6 5 4 3 2 1

Library of Congress Cataloging-in-Publication Data
Wedel, Johan, 1962–
Santería healing: a journey into the Afro-Cuban world of divinities,
spirits, and sorcery / Johan Wedel.
p. cm.—(Contemporary Cuba)
Includes bibliographical references (p.) and index.
ISBN 0-8130-2694-6 (c: alk. paper)
1. Santeria. 2. Spiritual healing—Cuba. 3. Healing—Religious
aspects—Santeria. 4. Medicine, Magic, mystic and spagiric—Cuba.
I. Title. II. Series.
BL2532.S3W43 2004
299.6'74'097291—dc22   2003061690

The University Press of Florida is the scholarly publishing agency
for the State University System of Florida, comprising Florida A&M
University, Florida Atlantic University, Florida Gulf Coast University,
Florida International University, Florida State University, University
of Central Florida, University of Florida, University of North Florida,
University of South Florida, and University of West Florida.

University Press of Florida
15 Northwest 15th Street
Gainesville, FL 32611-2079
http://www.upf.com

For Grédel

Contents

Figures and Tables

Figures

Tables

Foreword

Afro-Cuban religious expression has always been appealing, and also complex. It is reputed to be practiced by some 60–85 percent of the Cuban population (compared to the 2–3 percent who actively practice Catholicism). Some claim that Fidel Castro himself is an adherent. Significantly, Pope John Paul II refused to meet with leaders of Afro-Cuban religions when he visited Cuba in 1998, although he did meet with leaders of the Catholic, Jewish, and Protestant faiths. In the United States and, indeed, wherever Cuban communities are found, several forms of Afro-Cuban religious expression are practiced. The universality of this appeal is well illustrated by the fact that this book is written by a Swedish social anthropologist who mentions that even in Göteborg santería is practiced.

Unfortunately, Afro-Cuban religions are extremely difficult to penetrate for those not initiated in their belief systems. Johan Wedel is therefore to be commended for making available an insightful assessment of this integral facet of Cuban life and culture. In this book he offers an extremely useful history of the origins and evolution of santería, explains the basis for its wide appeal, and examines both its symbolism and its power in contemporary Cuba. He concludes with a useful critique of the current practice of Afro-Cuban religion in the "special period." The appendices, examining some technical areas of religious experience, are also worth noting. The focus on spiritual healing—the central thread of his analysis—is particularly helpful since it provides a well-argued illustration of the powers and attraction of this profoundly rooted religious expression. He also offers a useful interpretation of socially rooted medicine.

Santería is an area of Cuban life about which few have written so cogently, perhaps because Cubans are too close to it and writers with a Western superiority complex reject anything that could be viewed as "obscurantism." Wedel, by contrast, uses his natural curiosity and analytical skills to analyze and assess the religion. His findings shed a great deal of light on many areas of contemporary life in Cuba. The book is extremely useful for those seeking a general understanding of santería, as well as those interested in the medical anthropology of traditional medicine, Cuban style. Given the dearth of solid academic literature written on Afro-Cuban religious traditions, this study is particularly valuable.

The curiosity of the medical anthropologist is constantly noticeable, as Wedel pursues his pilgrimage of spiritual and medical exploration. In essence this is a process of demythification, as he seeks, successfully, to shed light onto the underpinnings of santería, its belief system, and its practice. Through a study of some hundred cases of religious-medical consultation with a local *santero*, Wedel is able to explore not only the value system inherent in this religious expression but also its widespread social appeal and medical value. Actual ceremonies, the divination process, the pantheon of *orishas* (gods), and the medical value of herbs employed are all painstakingly recreated by the curious medical anthropologist. Underlying this approach is the inherent comparison between contemporary biomedical curing techniques and traditional Afro-Cuban remedies (which maintain that illness is not located in the mind or body alone but also involves social relations and the individual's role within his or her community). This book studies an area of life directly or indirectly affecting most of the Cuban population, and in so doing, it allows us to penetrate an area of crucial importance that has long been overlooked. By laying aside Western prejudgments and examining Wedel's useful analysis, we can appreciate a driving force and essential component of the Cuban identity.

John M. Kirk
Series Editor

Preface

Although Cuba has a well-developed health care sector, many Cubans also seek help for their ailments from the Afro-Cuban religious tradition *santería*. Today it is increasingly common even for foreigners to come to Cuba and spend hundreds or thousands of dollars on initiations into santería because of illness. What is it that santería, with its roots in Africa and the slave trade, has to offer concerning illness and healing that Western medicine has not? Why have santería healing and its ideas about illness not disappeared in Cuba but instead flourished and even spread throughout the world? When I first visited Cuba in 1994, these were the questions that awakened my interest in santería, and they are the focus of this book.

In santería, illness is often understood as originating in disturbed social relations and sorcery. Healing implies developing relations with a spirit world manifested in mythology, divination systems, elaborate rituals, and nature itself. How can we make sense of such beliefs? I seek to give some answers to this question by examining how santería and its healing knowledge is practiced, experienced, and viewed in the climate of Cuba's current economic crisis. The book is based on fieldwork in Cuba and intended for an audience of scholars as well as others interested in santería, Cuba, and religious healing in general.

I wish to give warm thanks to all the people in Cuba who helped me with the study. In order to protect them, I have chosen not to mention their names. Parts of the book were originally presented as a Ph.D. dissertation at the Department of Social Anthropology, Göteborg University, Sweden, and I am especially grateful to the dissertation committee: Professor Roy Willis, Dr. Jan Bärmark, Dr. Ulla-Britt Engelbreksson, and Dr. Inger Sjørslev. Dr. Markel Thylefors has read several versions of the manuscript and given invaluable comments. I am deeply indebted to my tutor, Professor Kaj Århem, for his scholarly support and high standards. Warm thanks are also due to Dr. Alexandra Kent for carefully reading the manuscript. Additionally, I have benefited from the fact that several of my colleagues in the department are also working in the field of medical anthropology.

Parts of the manuscript were presented during various seminars at my department in Göteborg, and I wish to thank students, colleagues, and visiting professors for encouragement, comments, and moral support, especially Professor William Arens, Dr. Marita Eastmond, Bo Erntsson, Dr. Jan Hultin, Professor Bruce Kapferer, and Dr. Carola Skott. Earlier drafts of the chapters were presented at the workshop "Social og kulturell kreativitet på Cuba," University of Oslo, Norway (1997); at the conference "New African Perspectives: Africa, Australasia, and the Wider World at the End of the Twentieth Century," University of Western Australia, Perth, Australia (1999); and at the workshop "Medical Anthropology," University of Copenhagen, Copenhagen, Denmark (2000). I am grateful for the stimulating comments and criticism I received on these and other occasions. Thanks also to series editor John Kirk, to Amy Gorelick at the University Press of Florida, and to George Brandon and Mary Ann Clark for helpful comments in the final stages of writing the book.

I would also like to acknowledge the financial support received from the Swedish Institute, Helge Ax:son Johnsons Stiftelse, Svenska Sällskapet för Antropologi och Geografi, Adlerbertska forskningsfonden, and Swedish International Development Cooperation Agency/Department for Research Cooperation. Finally, I am particularly grateful to my wife Grédel for her encouragement and comments, and I dedicate this book to her.

Introduction

On the seventeenth day of December, 1997, the feastday of San Lazaro, a priest of the Afro-Cuban religious tradition santería walks from central Havana to the small village of El Rincón and the Church of San Lazaro, a distance of more than thirty kilometers. Many others do the same. Pilgrims come in buses, cars, and horse-drawn vehicles. Some ride bicycles or arrive on foot, and they come from all over Cuba. A short distance from the church on both sides of the road, people are selling grilled meat and lemonade. A few are sitting with a statue of San Lazaro and a small box into which passersby throw coins.

The crowd on the road sometimes makes way for pilgrims edging their way toward the church. With their clothes torn to pieces and covered with dirt, they are close to fainting in the morning heat. They have made vows in order to be helped by the saint and are now fulfilling their part of the promise. When the pilgrims finally enter the crowded church, they throw themselves in front of one of the altars of San Lazaro. All the time more people arrive. Some of them walk on their knees. The floor is covered with lit candles, flowers, and eggs that people have used to "cleanse" themselves from bad influences and sorcery. The crowd carefully avoids stepping on the eggs. A thin man in his early thirties from the AIDS clinic nearby sits on the floor with a puppy and a miniature statue of San Lazaro in his hands. The santería priest from central Havana greets him and throws a coin on the floor in front of him.

The pilgrimage to the Church of San Lazaro can be considered a Roman Catholic event, but from the point of view of those who practice santería, it is also a way to pay respect to, and ask for help from, an important divinity of the santería pantheon of *orishas*. San Lazaro, or Babalú Ayé as he also is called, is the great healer of illness in santería. There are many stories of people who have been miraculously healed by him.

Santería, la Regla de Ocha ("the way of the saints"), is a practical, adaptive, and holistic religious tradition. It aims at well-being and for the resolution of problems in this world, here and now. When its followers are confronted with sickness or misfortune, they will not only ask *how* it happened but also *why*. Frequently, this is done by relating sickness to the ill person's social relations and way of life and to the santería world of spirits and divinities. It is not enough to look for a cure if the underlying causes of the problem have not been identified. For the followers of santería, sickness can be avoided and health achieved through rituals and initiations, and by offerings and sacrifices to the santería divinities. In this way, humans are empowered in their daily life and protected against supernatural forces.

Santería has its roots in Africa and the slave trade, when many slaves were taken to Cuba. A considerable number of these were Yoruba, from present-day Nigeria, who worshipped divinities known as orishas. The religious beliefs of the Yoruba slaves were reconstituted in Cuba within a new social framework that gave rise to the santería religion, which, in the process, was influenced by Roman Catholicism. Today, a large portion of the Cuban population practices santería. As an important part of modern life, it is visible in both the public and the private spheres. Followers of santería greatly outnumber practicing Protestants and Jews and adherents of the Roman Catholic Church, which was relatively weak before the revolution and remained so after it.

A few days after the pilgrimage, in a large plaza in front of the sea in Havana, thousands of people listen and dance to Paulito y Su Élite, one of the most popular salsa music groups. Paulito, himself a santería initiate, shouts: "Raise your hands, children of Shangó," and then "Raise your hands, children of Obatalá, . . . Yemayá, . . . Ogún."[1] The audience shouts and people raise their hands when the santería divinity with whom they identify is mentioned. The close relation to the orishas is also expressed in another salsa music concert sometime later when the group Adalberto y Su Son sings: "He who messes with me, messes with Shangó."

Not everyone in Cuba is a santería devotee, but the idea that every person is protected and related to a certain santería divinity (orisha or *santo*) is widespread. Santo is the Spanish word for the Roman Catholic "saint," but it also means orisha in the Afro-Cuban context. I will use santo instead of orisha when referring to the divinities of the santería pantheon, because santo is the term most frequently used in Cuba. It is by gradually developing a relationship with the santos that one can gain all kinds of help, be given protection, and be healed from illness. On the streets all over Cuba it is common to see people who have created a deep relationship with the santos by being

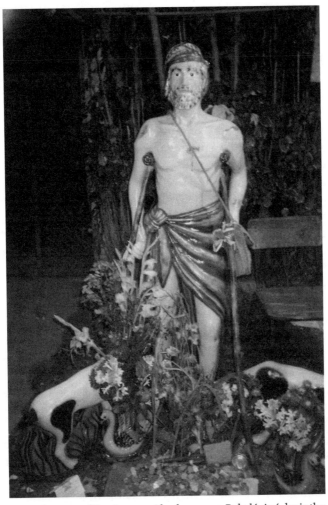

Fig. 1. A statue of San Lazaro. Also known as Babalú Ayé, he is the lord of skin ailments and infectious diseases but also the great healer of illness. Photo by Johan Wedel.

initiated. They wear white clothes and headdresses, and necklaces and bracelets that, through their combinations of colors, refer to a certain santo. The colorful beaded necklaces can be found at the marketplace, in stores, and at the *yerbero* (the herbalist), where objects representing the santería divinities are available for purchase.

In a large store on the main street in Matanzas, all kinds of Cuban-made goods are sold: furniture, underwear, cosmetics, textiles, buckets, kitchenware, and so on. There is even a cafeteria. Santería artifacts are sold at one counter. One can find pulverized eggshells, butter from cacao and palm nut, ceramic soup tureens, beaded necklaces, a small cauldron with miniature iron tools, a miniature bow and arrow, and an iron bird on a dowel. These iron artifacts represent the three "warriors": Ogún, lord of iron, war, and hard work; Ochosi, the divine hunter; and Ósun, protector and guardian. They are placed behind the front door of the devotee's house together with a "head," usually made of stone or cement, often with eyes and mouth made of cowrie shells. This is Eleggua, the messenger, trickster, and guardian of crossroads.

Being involved in santería means coming under the protection of the divine world of the santos, and an initiated devotee is called *santera* (female) or *santero* (male). Involvement in santería also implies social obligations and obligations to the divinities, and new perspectives on the world. This, in turn, is closely related to the fact that many seek help from the santos, and possibly become initiates, in order to resolve problems of ill health. This is not to say that there are no other reasons for becoming involved in the religion; many turn to santería with financial or legal problems. Others have family members who are santería priests and find it natural to become part of the religious practice of their families. Issues concerning sickness and health, however, are one of the most, if not *the* most prominent theme, when people explain why they consult a santería priest or become initiated.

Santería is today a religious tradition of significance in Cuba. Its rituals include divination, sacrifice, possession trance, and herbal medicine, and it emphasizes the meaningful and transcendent experience of illness. Healing in santería is dependent on the form of sickness and its underlying causes, the afflicted person's relations to humans, spirits, and divinities, and the knowledge of the santería priest. The view of ill health and its causes is radically different from the Western biomedical view. My aim, then, is to develop an understanding of how santería healing works, how it is carried out, and how it is experienced. The study, which is also intended as a contribution to the study of religious healing in general, is grounded in an account of how individuals experience healing and how they live through illness. This also implies an examination of the "systems of classification that we may trace behind diagnosis and treatment" (Jacobson-Widding 1989:15), but the focus is on individual experience.

The present work is, to my knowledge, one of very few studies in English based on social anthropological fieldwork in Cuba. The only other major works to date are Lewis et al. (1977a, 1977b, 1978); Butterworth (1974, 1980); Daniel (1995); and Rosendahl (1997a, 1997b). None of these, however, focuses on santería. There exist several works about santería that are either general accounts or studies based on its practices in the United States (e.g., Murphy 1993; Brandon 1993; Curry 1997; Sandoval 1977, 1979; Jones et al. 2001; Pasquali 1986, 1994). The studies of santería as it is practiced in Cuba today are based on research in Cuba but are generally descriptive, lack anthropological analysis, and are written in Spanish (e.g., Cabrera 1993a; Bolívar 1990; Guanche 1983). Three exceptions are Palmié (2002), Dianteill (2000), and Hagedorn (2001). These works are based on anthropological fieldwork in Cuba carried out during the 1990s; the first focuses on modernity and tradition, the second on initiation and written sources, and the third on performance. The present work is also, as far as I know, the first study that focuses on the healing and illness aspects of santería on the island, despite the central role given to these issues.

Inspired by three important anthropological works on religious healing from different parts of the world (Csordas 1994; Friedson 1996; Willis 1999), I examine how santería healing is experienced and attempt to show that santería healing is best understood as a transformation of the self in which the ill person begins to experience the world in new ways. This is the case particularly during the week-long initiation when a "remaking" of the world takes place; the initiate will encounter, develop relations to, and embrace, the otherworld of divinities and spirits. In relation to this, I show that santería healing is, to a large extent, an open-ended process dependent on the behavior of the person being healed and based on a relationship between humans and divinities.

When someone decides to become initiated into santería, that person begins to develop a new sense of the self. If initiation is carried out, he or she will not only begin to think and act differently but also to feel differently. Gradually, the ill person comes to experience the world in a deeply religious way. He begins to understand illness from a new perspective; body and mind, self and other begin to interpenetrate in new ways. This transformation of the self and reorientation toward the world is an important part of what constitutes healing in santería. In order to understand santería healing, then, it is not sufficient to explore its symbols and its meaning; it is also necessary to understand how healing is experienced by those who suffer from illness, undergo initiation or some minor ritual, and are healed.

The present study is written in a phenomenological tradition within anthropology that emphasizes embodied experience and narratives. In this tradition, understanding a healing ritual, for example, involves inquiring into how healing is experienced from within: how it affects the participants; how ritual performance may change how people feel; and how they become existentially engaged in the process (Desjarlais 1992; Csordas 1996; Laderman and Roseman 1996).

This approach focuses on particular men and women in particular situations and on their interpretation of their own practices (Kleinman 1995). From this perspective, it becomes important to examine what different beliefs accomplish for those who invoke and use them. Lived experience is privileged over theoretical knowledge in order to explore the existential uses and consequences of beliefs, and to tell ordinary people's stories in their own words (Jackson 1996). Through people's stories we "move away from excessive abstraction and ground one's discourse in the sentient life of individuals interacting with objects and with others in the quotidian world" (Jackson 1989:18). Through the stories people tell about themselves and others around them, we learn about experience.

Narratives are stories about lived experience and are therefore central to an understanding of illness and healing. They provide a point of entry into the life world of people's experiences, and they place events in a meaningful order in time. Narratives also place illness and healing in relation to a larger whole, to other events in life. Hence, we should not restrict ourselves to a description of what illness or healing "feels like." The aim is to "focus on how dimensions of the perceived world are 'unmade,' broken down or altered, as a result of serious illness, as well as on the restitutive processes of the 'remaking' of the world" (Good 1994:131).

My analytical tools and my examination of santería healing are based on medical anthropology, a subdiscipline of anthropology. Medical anthropology critically examines Western medical beliefs and studies how people around the world respond to sickness. Instead of taking the Western biomedical view of sickness and curing for granted, medical anthropology views biomedicine (Western medicine) as one cultural system among many others. By studying both Western and non-Western ideas of sickness and curing/healing, medical anthropology aims to expand "Western ideas about humanity [and] . . . to promote mutual respect, communication across boundaries, and exchange where it may be beneficial" (Hahn 1995:2).

In medical anthropology, a useful distinction between two aspects of sickness is often made: the distinction between disease and illness. These concepts were developed and discussed by Kleinman (1980) and later by Finkler (1994) and others. I seek to follow this dichotomy and view disease as a malfunctioning related to biological and biochemical processes in the body. Disease primarily belongs to biomedicine while illness is about "the whole experience of being unwell" (Strathern and Stewart 1999:6). Illness refers to cultural meanings and experience, and to the social environment as a possible source of an affliction. It is important to recognize that these are overlapping concepts, not separate entities, developed in order to gain a broader understanding of sickness.

Following this dichotomy I will also use the distinction between curing and healing. Curing belongs mainly to biomedicine and refers to the successful treatment of a specific condition, such as an infection or a broken leg. Healing, on the other hand, refers to personal experience and the whole person in relation to other components in life. Healing depends on personal experience and satisfaction with treatment. These concepts also overlap: a person may become cured while being healed.

As a starting point, I introduce in the first chapter two santería devotees and their families. The two women, whom I call Matilda and Eva, have struggled against malady for long periods, and both have experienced relief and healing through santería. The presentation is intended to give a first experience-near account of santería healing. During the course of the book, the two women's beliefs and responses to illness will be elucidated and given deeper meaning.

In chapter 2 I present a historical account of the formation of santería (from the time of slavery to the present time of the economic crisis). I trace the role of santería as a means of healing and briefly discuss santería's role in the larger historical processes in Cuban society. I also explore the recent economic crisis in Cuba in relation to santería. Many who suffer the consequences of the economic crisis, and experience a situation that is both capricious and uncertain, find relief and solution to their problems through santería.

Chapter 3 focuses on the perceived relations between human beings and divinities, and the meaning of life force *(ashé)*. Possible causes of illness are examined, especially divine "punishment," afflicting spirits, and sorcery. The focus then shifts to an examination of common responses to illness through santería. The roles of sacrifice, beauty, music, dance, and possession trance in healing are discussed, as are the reshaping of social relations through involvement in santería. Finally, I inquire into the use of herbs and plants in healing.

In chapter 4 I examine the pantheon and rituals within which santería and its ideas about healing and illness are inscribed. I give a presentation of the orishas/santos and their characteristics and give some examples from the rich santería mythology. I also discuss santería rituals, including divination, and give an account of the initiation, which is a week-long ceremony that brings about a profound change in the initiate's life.

Chapter 5 examines santería healing from a more general comparative point of view. A discussion of santería ontology and self suggests that mind, body, and social relations are interwoven with each other. The importance of nature in santería, and how nature achieves a new and divine meaning for the initiate, is also discussed. Finally, santería healing is compared with biomedical curing, and the relation between these two systems is examined.

Chapter 6 focuses on narratives about illness and healing in order to give a more profound understanding of how people relate to the divinities and experience healing. These cases show how the narrators acquire, in their own perception, a broader understanding of illness that includes both social relations and relations to the otherworld of spirits and divinities. The stories also show how relations to the otherworld are developed and nurtured over time in order to both restore and maintain health.

In chapter 7 I take a closer look at some of the criticisms of santería and give voice to people who are skeptical of santería practice. The critique is often related to the economic crisis, and it is claimed that many santería priests exploit people and take advantage of their difficult situation. Finally, in chapter 8 the argument and its implications are summed up.

Research was conducted in Cuba over fifteen months between 1996 and 2001. I used the anthropological qualitative-research strategy known as participant observation. This implies documenting complex details of everyday life over a long period of time, living among ordinary people and speaking the local language. The method relies partly on interviews. Of equal importance, however, is participation and observation of actual behavior since people will often say one thing but think and do something else.

Part of the time I was affiliated as a postgraduate student at the University of Havana. During my stay, I participated in seminars and two postgraduate courses in anthropology. The courses included fieldwork, and several of my interviews were made while taking part in the courses. I also studied the Spanish language at the university, and, while improving my Spanish inside and outside class, I learned about various aspects of Cuban history and society. At the time, Cuba was suffering deeply from an economic crisis that began after the Soviet bloc collapsed. I worked in Havana and in Matanzas, a city located about one hundred kilometers east of Havana. Despite their difficult economic situation I found people extremely helpful and friendly, and I was able to interview a number of people who had some kind of relation to santería. I took part in and witnessed several dozen rituals, from large initiation ceremonies to spiritual baths and divination sessions.

As I gradually entered into a world where invisible, magical forces were seen as real and tangible, and where spirits and divinities made their presence felt not only in rituals but also in daily life, I began to see things from the point of view of a santería follower. In this perception of the world, it made perfect sense to counter illness and misfortune with offerings, sacrifices, music, and possession trance. On several occasions I was spiritually "cleansed," and I carried out sacrifices that had been prescribed during divination sessions. I did not, however, become initiated, and I never experienced any altered state of consciousness during drum rituals (although I felt more calm and empowered after performing the so-called "rogation of the head" ritual).

Despite this lack of any profound experience with the otherworld, my encounter with santería became a kind of spiritual journey as I began to think differently about things I had not previously questioned. Communication with the divine through divination and possession trance, and the way people experienced illness as resulting from acts of sorcery, made me question how we in the West think about the self in relation to other humans and to the world around us. Santería made me understand that the Western distinction between mind and body is not as clear and obvious as we often think and that social relations are imperative when understanding the process behind healing and illness.

Extended interviews were carried out with more than twenty santería priests, their clients, and others related to santería and with several followers of the religious traditions *espiritismo* and *palo monte*. My main informant in Matanzas was a santería priest who also practiced palo monte and espiritismo. In Havana, some of my informants were *babalaos*, high priests who work with the Ifá divination system, and two of them were also physicians.

I chose Matanzas as my field site as this city is known for being a place where santería is "well preserved." Many outsiders, both from different parts of Cuba and from abroad, come to the city to be initiated. Many who go through initiation also visit Havana, but here the religion is becoming more commercialized. In Havana there are also more expressions of santería outside of its religious context. I found minor differences in the performance of rituals, but the ways people experienced santería and the manners of healing were similar in the two cities. In order to protect informants, their names have been fictionalized.

I

❦❦❦

The Struggle against Illness

Matilda and Her Family

In a backyard in Matanzas, a group of people stand in silence around a hole in the ground. A santería priest begins to pass a white rooster over their bodies, one after the other. He cuts the throat of the bird, and the blood pours down into the hole. The participants also "cleanse" themselves with all kinds of vegetables and beans. The fowl, beans, and vegetables are then thrown into the hole, which is finally covered with earth. Matilda and her relatives are giving "food to the earth."

Matilda, a woman in her early fifties who has been a santera for fourteen years, explains: "We are doing this because there is sickness in the family. Some time ago, one of my aunts died of illness, then an uncle, then a cousin of my sister. My mother died very recently. When I went for a [santería] consultation, a *letra* [a divination sign] came up that spoke about sickness, and it said that we had to give *comida para la tierra* [food to the earth] in order to give health to everyone. It's a very strong letra so everybody has to be present. This is very important for my husband and myself because we are both sick."

According to the santero who performed the ceremony, one gives food to the earth when someone is very ill and about to die: "When one is sick, the earth is calling. You give food to the earth so that the earth will eat this food and not eat you. One sacrifices and buries different kinds of food and animals such as a chicken, a rooster, a pigeon, or what the earth wants, in order to cover the hole of illness and death."

Matilda lives with her husband Oscar in one of the poorest neighbor-hoods of Matanzas. Houses in this area are generally small and crowded. During the rainy season the streets get flooded and muddy water enters the houses. Long power outages are common, especially when it is raining. Many who live here are unemployed, and the inhabitants have a reputation for involvement in illegal activities. But the neighborhood is also famous for its many skilled rumba musicians and santería practitioners. The majority are people with an African heritage. On the streets at night, it is common to hear song and the sound of drums from a santería ritual.

Matilda and Oscar have a small concrete house they built themselves. The living room is sparsely furnished. An old sofa, a black-and-white TV, and a broken wooden chair take up most of the room. Matilda shows her own and Oscar's santería objects, which are hidden behind a curtain. On a wall above the objects hangs a machete. "It's for [the divinity] Ogún," she says. Outside, a pig and some chickens walk around freely in the muddy yard that belongs to the house. Matilda has two daughters and one son. Her oldest daughter, Florencia, who herself had a child about a year ago, also lives in the house. When Matilda decided to become initiated, she was suf-fering from severe pain in her belly:

I had a lot of pain in my belly and went to many different doctors. They always had different opinions about my problem. One said it was a cyst, another said it was a small tumor, another said another thing. My mother, who is a santera, said it was because of sorcery. She said I had been given something "bad" to eat or drink. I didn't want to be oper-ated on. Finally I did it but nothing changed, I still had pain.

During that time, I didn't believe much in santería and I never went to santería parties, but I went to a santero for him to *mirarme*, "look at me" [divine]. He told me that I had to "make santo" [become initiated into santería] and that my son and husband also had to do it, in order to avoid illness. In my husband's family there is madness. In order not to become mad, he had to make santo. The three of us made santo together. I made [became initiated and related to the divinity] Yemayá, my son made Shangó, and my husband made Ogún.

The seven days in the *cuarto de santo* (initiation room) was a very special experience. I slept on the floor the whole time, something I never thought I would do. People took very good care of me, like a child. They gave me food, and every morning I drank *omiero* [herbal medicine]. During the divination [performed during initiation], I was promised that I would not have any more problems with my belly. On the fourth day, I made the "presentation" [ritually danced and paid tribute to the santería sacred drums]. I danced, but the santo did not "descend" on me, and to this day I have never become possessed.

Over the following year, I slowly began to feel a little better. I knew that I would not get well directly. It is a slow process. I drank herbal medicine and did cleansings and baths. I was prohibited from eating eggs, animal heads and offal, canned meat, and calabash. All these prohibitions were related to the problem I had. If I eat any of these things, in one minute I will be affected. Today I also sometimes take herbal medicine. My father-in-law is a *palero* [priest of the religious tradition palo monte] and also knows about herbs. When I want to cleanse my house or myself, I ask him which herb to use. If, for example, I have a problem with my husband, there is an herb for that, too.

Today, Matilda often participates in santería ceremonies and dances in drum feasts when she is invited. She especially likes the *tambor para egún* (drum ceremony for the dead): "In the ceremony the santo 'descends' [possesses a devotee] and cleanses people and gives them advice about what to do and not do." Although she is largely positive about santería, she complains that it has become very expensive to perform any kind of "work." Despite this, she claims that her two daughters have to become initiated sooner or later: "It's like a chain; when someone in the family makes santo, the others also have to do it. My daughters have to make santo in order to protect themselves. I am protected from sorcery, but if someone performs sorcery on me, my daughters or anybody else who lives in the house may catch it and become ill or die because they are not protected."

A few weeks after the family gave food to the earth, Matilda once again performs a ritual, but this time the rest of her family does not participate. She brings a surgical knife and needle, a small goat, a chicken, and some of her clothing that contains her sweat. The babalao who is in charge of the ceremony cleanses her with the surgical instruments and sacrifices the animals. He then makes a packet of everything and instructs Matilda to bring it to the cemetery and leave it there.

According to Matilda, the ritual is performed in order to avoid an operation: "I do this *ebbó* [sacrifice] because I have problems with gallstones or my kidneys, and I have a lot of pain in the mornings. I work in a store, and when I lift anything, it hurts. I have been seeing a doctor for a long time and have received injections. But the doctor is not sure of what it is because I don't have any of the ordinary symptoms, and my urine is normal."

The last time Matilda went to the physician, she was told that she had to be operated upon. She became frightened and went to a santería priest for a consultation: "Eleggua told me [through divination] that if I made a sacrifice [ebbó] I would not have to undergo an operation. To be sure I also went to a babalao, which is the highest person in this religion; he has the final word. He consulted Orula, who also told me to wait. The babalao told me to make a beverage from zapote leaves [see app. 1] and drink it for seven days, three times a day, and then do the ebbó. Now I will go to the doctor again and see if the operation is still necessary, or if I can avoid it."

Matilda's Husband, Oscar

In a colonial house in the old part of Matanzas, a drum ceremony is taking place. More than forty people have gathered in a small room, and the sound of drums attracts neighbors and passersby. Matilda's husband, Oscar, is one of the participants. He is in the middle of the crowd, watching how people dance in front of the sacred drums. Suddenly, he begins to shake furiously. He bends his body back and forth and almost falls to the ground. Two people help him to stand straight. Then, he becomes calm and begins to dance to the music. The divinity Ogún has temporarily descended and possessed Oscar's body. He is given a machete that he swings in the air while smoking a cigar.

The following morning I talked with Oscar about what had happened. "Ogún is my father," Oscar said, and continued: "People say that I become possessed with Ogún. When he descends it's not me anymore. When he mounts, he is the owner of my person. It's not the same person, it's Ogún. I am far away. People also tell me that when Ogún 'comes down,' he swings a machete, smokes cigars, and speaks *Lucumí* [the santería ritual language]. I don't understand Lucumí, and I don't like to smoke, but Ogún does. He also likes blood from dogs, so there should be no dogs around when he is present. He may bite and kill them. Ogún is violent, but he may also sit in a chair and advise people. When he leaves I always have a headache, so I don't go very often to drum feasts."

Sometimes, Oscar becomes possessed with Ogún when he is sleeping, walking the streets, or riding a bicycle. "When this happens in the street, one must find someone who understands and speaks Lucumí," he says. Lucumí is a creolized form of the Yoruba language, spoken by the santería divinities when they possess a devotee. If Oscar becomes possessed in the neighborhood and someone knows where he lives, he is taken home. Ogún is then given a machete, dressed in a rustic piece of gray cloth that Oscar keeps in the house, and asked why he has descended: "Often, Ogún comes down because he wants to warn someone of a danger or illness. It may be that Ogún has a message for someone who is ill, someone who must change his *camino* [way] in life or else something bad will happen. It's in order to say that here is a danger that the person doesn't know about."

When Oscar became initiated fourteen years ago (together with his wife and their son), he had a stomach ulcer. A doctor explained that his problem was related to his drinking habits, and Oscar was given different medications: "At that time my life was crazy. I drank heavily and lived in different places. When I made santo, all that changed. During the *itá* [divination] I was told to stop drinking, or I would die. I was also forbidden to eat calabash and colored beans, which affected my stomach. My wife also changed very much after she made santo. Before, she had many problems, but today she is very calm. She is protected by her santos. Now she is doing a sacrifice because of illness. I also have to do a cleansing for my health."

According to Oscar, sorcery is very common in the neighborhood he lives in, and many palo monte practitioners perform evil sorcery.[1] "It's very dangerous," he says. "It can even kill the sorcerer himself." If Oscar, or someone in his family, becomes ill and he suspects sorcery, he often consults his father, who is a palero. Oscar's father knows about sorcery protection and can identify the evildoer. Oscar is well protected against sorcery both because he is a santero and because he practices the religious tradition espiritismo:

> I can feel in my body when something bad is going to happen. When someone is about to perform sorcery on me and my family, I dream that sorcery is coming. Then I tell my wife. I have to tell her quickly so we can prepare ourselves. The *muertos* [spirits of the dead] also help me. I practice spiritism and have a *bóveda* [spiritist table], and the dead come to me a lot. They don't leave me alone. They caress my feet when I am sleeping, but they don't want anything bad. If it was bad, the whole house would be upside down. They do it in order to tell me something, to warn me. If I want the spirits to leave me alone and not disturb me, I get up and put some *cascarilla* [pulverized eggshells] and perfume on my feet. My wife doesn't like that, and she doesn't work with the dead. I think it's because she is afraid, that's the problem.

Matilda's Daughter Florencia

Florencia, Matilda's oldest child, is about twenty-five years old. She holds a degree from the University of Matanzas in engineering but works as a cleaning lady in a large hotel in the nearby tourist resort Varadero. "A normal monthly salary for an engineer is less than four hundred pesos (twenty dollars). I make more money from the tips in the hotel than I would ever do as an engineer. Here it does not matter that you have a university degree. In this country we are completely dependent on tourism," she says.

Florencia does not practice santería and is skeptical about her parents' beliefs and santería's ability to resolve illness problems: "I am really not much of a believer. My mother has her way to believe, and she has not had any serious illness problem since she made santo. But I don't think it's because of the santos. It's something psychological. It's inside her, like, 'I made santo and I'm okay.' It's only her thoughts. If you have a positive attitude, everything will turn out well. If you think negative and carry a negative influence, it will go wrong." Despite her skepticism, Florencia has performed santería rituals and participated in spiritist masses. She does not exclude the possibility that she may become initiated one day:

I think I will make santo because everybody in my family is religious, and everybody has made santo except my daughter, my sister, my niece, and myself. When I was pregnant, my mother told me all the time to pass a calabash over my belly. In the end I finally did it, and everything went well. My mother also went to a santero and did some work when my sister was in jail. She got out and everything went well. But that has not really made me believe. If something happens to my daughter and some work is done that gives a good result, then I will believe more. If I see it with my own eyes. I believe more in the existence of sorcery and in the spirits [of the dead]. I have been to [spiritist] masses where spirits possess people and they transform completely. They do *rompimiento* [ritual against evil influences] and take away *muertos oscuros* [dark spirits] from people who are ill. The spirit gives the name and address of the person who performed the sorcery, and says why.

Florencia does not agree with her parents about the dangers of sorcery. "I don't think I have to protect myself. If I haven't done any harm to anybody, nothing will happen to me," she says. She is also reluctant to become involved in santería for financial reasons:

You may be desperate, seriously ill, and about to die. Then, the priest says: "With this and this you will resolve your problem." It's a lie. When you are destined to die, you die. With or without santo. If there is no cure it's better for the family to spend the money on something other than santería. There are santeros who will exploit you. If a piece

of bread that you pass over your body is sufficient to resolve your problem, then why does the santero have to say, "Bring me two goats, bring
me two pigeons, bring me a hen"? It's exploitation, and you see it often
in the countryside where santeros even fool the peasants to sacrifice
pigs, but pigs have nothing to do with santería.

Eva and Her Family

Eva lives with her husband and daughter in a newly developed area of small
family houses outside Matanzas. Her house, built about twenty years ago, is
a one-story concrete building with four rooms and a yard at the back. It is a
peaceful place, and some of the neighbors' children play on the dusty street
in front of the house. The street was never sealed with asphalt despite plans
to do so. As with many building projects, the development of the area came
to a halt when the economic crisis, the so-called special period, began in
1990.

Three months ago, Eva became initiated into santería after a long period
of suffering and illness. Today she will begin the ritual known as the *ebbó de
tres meses* (three-months' sacrifice). The santero Máximo, who is Eva's godfather, has invited me to participate, and we are going with his daughter and a
friend. As we cruise out of Matanzas in an old Ford, trying to close the back
door and hold still the two fowls we have brought with us, Máximo points at
a goat on the roadside. "With one of these, all your problems would be
solved," he says to his daughter. She has financial problems and often fights
and argues with her mother. According to her father, the sacrifice of a goat
would bring an end to her problems.

When we arrive at Eva's house, she runs out to welcome us. One of the
latest salsa songs by Los Van Van is playing loudly from one of the bedrooms: "Be careful, be careful, we are Negroes Lucumí." Eva is about forty-
five years old and very energetic. She is an *iyabó* (new initiate); her long
black hair is covered with a white headdress, and she wears a white dress
with beaded necklaces in different colors. In the garden in front of the
house, a fifty-year-old Chevrolet without windows is parked, surrounded by
motor parts. A goat and a sheep are tied to the car. They will be sacrificed
later.

In the yard at the back of the house, there are cages with pigeons, cockerels, hens, ducks, and a turkey. They will also be sacrificed during the ceremony. I count sixteen fowls, excluding the pigeons. Three elderly santeras,
who will help the santero and participate in the ceremony, have already ar-

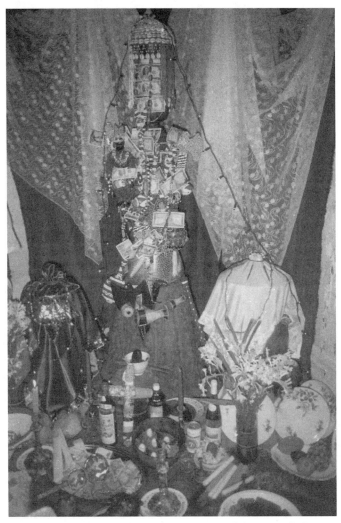

Fig. 2. Santería altars. The owner is a powerful priest of Shangó, which can be seen by the large, expensive altar of Shangó in the middle. Photo by Johan Wedel.

rived. As we sit down and gossip about other santería devotees and possible cases of sorcery, Eva's husband gives us bad news: eleven white pigeons have escaped. The sacrifice cannot begin until they are found. Two boys with slingshots are sent out to find them. Meanwhile, more people arrive. Some are godchildren to Eva's new santería godfather Máximo, and therefore also her new "brothers" and "sisters," while others are friends and neighbors. By early afternoon, the two boys have managed to capture some of the pigeons. Fortunately, a neighbor gives Eva the rest, and the ceremony can begin.

A short ceremony for the dead ancestors is first performed at a small altar with flowers and glasses of water in the backyard. Máximo prays and hits the ground with a stick. The dead are offered maize, sugar, and honey on a plate. Two pigeons are sacrificed, and the santero divines with coconut shells in order to make sure that the dead are pleased. The ceremony for the dead ends with a Catholic prayer. It is now time to prepare the omiero and to wash all the ritual objects in the liquid. The ceremony, which takes place in Eva's bedroom, is secret, and only santería initiates participate. The door is closed, but I can hear them singing inside in Lucumí. When they are ready, Eva's godfather divines again with four pieces of coconut. Everything will turn out well, but he says that Eva worries too much and must be more relaxed.

The sacrifice is to be performed in the living room. The goat, the sheep, and two roosters are brought in. Eva's objects representing the divinities Ogún and Eleggua are placed in the middle of the room. Eva is first cleansed with the fowls. They are then sacrificed together with the sheep and the goat. The blood pours over the objects as everybody sings in Lucumí, and everything is finally covered with feathers.

The procedure is repeated until all of Eva's santos have "eaten." Throughout the whole process, the santero has been divining with the coconut shells and has "asked" each santo about Eva's relation to divinities, humans, and spirits. When the first day of the three-day ceremony is over, part of the meat is distributed among the participants. Tomorrow, Eva will perform a ceremony directed at peace and stability called "rogation of the head" *(rogación de cabeza)*, and on the third day a more profound divination will take place.

Eva has struggled against serious illness and other problems for many years, and santería has come to play an important role in that battle. Her problems began when she got married for the first time: "I had a normal childhood. I often went to the church with my mother, and this has given me a strong Catholic faith. When I was twenty I got married, but almost at once I began to have problems with my husband. He hit me and treated me very badly. I suffered so much that I decided to take my life. In order to burn myself, I put alcohol on my body in the bathroom and locked the door. My neighbor broke the door and took me out. My clothes were on fire but I did not burn myself. It was incredible that I survived."

After awhile Eva married again and lived a tranquil life for a few years. At the time, she did not know anything about santería or spiritism. "That did not exist in my family," she says. By the time she was thirty years old, Eva had separated again, and then she met her present husband. At this time her health problems returned. First, she had a lump on her breast that she thought was cancer. She had a cytological test that showed she did not have cancer, but Eva was worried. A few years later, a more detailed examination showed that she now had cancer, and because Eva's mother and sister had died young of cancer of the uterus, the doctors told her to have an operation. Eva also became pregnant with her second child.

> I was six months pregnant. One doctor told me that I had to do an urgent operation and interrupt the pregnancy. He said, "If we don't operate, you will die and leave your child without a mother." My husband and I went back from the hospital crying. It was very hard for us that we were going to lose the child. Then something strange happened. A few days before the operation I was sitting under a tree in my backyard talking to a neighbor. Suddenly, a one-meter-long serpent fell down on my neck. I grabbed it with both hands and threw it away, and it disappeared into the bush. I was very frightened and peed in my pants. Later I understood what it meant; I was cleansed with the serpent.
>
> When my husband went back to the hospital, the doctors had changed their minds and said that it was better to wait with the operation. Everything went well with the pregnancy, but after I had my child I went through the operation and all my reproductive organs were removed. I was thirty-three and would never menstruate again.

Two years later, Eva faced an even more serious health problem when she had a heart attack:

> I came to the hospital with a lot of pain, and it took some time before the doctors understood what it was. I had an infarct and my heart was in a very bad condition. I was dying. They gave me a lot of medicine and told me I had less than three months to live. I was sent to a hospital in Havana, and the head of the cardiology department said that I could not undergo an operation because my heart was too damaged. He said, "We can't spend resources on an operation because you will not survive. We can't do anything." I began to cry and said to the doctor, "I have my daughter and I want to live for her. She needs me, you must do something."

Eva was given all kinds of medicine. The doctor told her to go back home, but he also promised that he would try to find a solution. Sometime later Eva underwent the operation. When she was sent home, Eva was in a very bad condition. At the time, she was beginning to feel a strange sensation in her body:

> I began to have symptoms that were not normal. It wasn't pain. My feet became cold, and this coldness went up and I felt emptiness in my stomach, like my life was leaving me. I cried because I thought I was going to die. I would rise and walk around to make it go away. Later I understood that it was [the divinity] Obatalá telling me something.
>
> One day a friend of mine came by and said, "Why don't you go and see someone who is religious in order to see if you can become better?" I said, "I don't believe in that, I only believe in God. These are demonic things of the devil." She insisted, "Go and see someone." I felt so sick, I was at the point of dying, so I said, "Okay, I will go with you." I was taken to a married couple who were sorcerers. I was given necklaces, [objects of the divinity] Olokun, and I was cleansed with some sticks.
>
> After that I became much worse. They almost finished me off completely. They were palo monte priests, paleros, and not santeros, but despite that, they were giving me things of santería. Everything went very bad. I had to go back to the hospital, the household economy broke down, I wanted to kill myself, and my husband almost brought me to a psychiatrist.

At the time, Eva was running a small café with her husband, but their small business was heavily taxed. In addition, questions were being raised as to whether they had illegally acquired the ingredients for making cakes and sweets. Finally they had to close down. For Eva, this was bad luck caused by the palo monte priests that, together with her health situation, made life very difficult. Despite her bad experience with religious experts, Eva felt that she had no other choice but to continue to search for someone who could help her.

After a short time, Eva's husband brought her to a santera and she was cleansed with herbs: "I didn't want to do anything against God, but I was very ill and thought, 'Well, there is always the possibility this might help.' I wanted to live. I began to visit the santera and received [santería] necklaces, and, miraculously, I became better. The santera told me, 'You were born to become a queen, you have to be crowned.' She did not consult with the shells, but she told me to visit another santero in order to divine which santo I had to make."

Eva found a santero who divined and told her that she was very ill and could die at any moment. She had to do a *medio asiento* (a halfway initiation) as soon as possible. Eva went through the ceremony, and the santero became her godfather. It was expensive, but because Eva's daughter lives in the United States and sometimes sends money, she could afford it. She received the objects representing the divinity Eleggua and the warriors and then the objects of the divinity Oyá. To "receive" means to create a relation between the individual and a certain divinity. A profound divination was performed during the halfway initiation, and Eva was told that she also had to perform a complete initiation and make Oyá. She began to prepare for the ceremony but had a feeling that something was wrong:

> Some of the animals I bought for the ceremony died, and I felt that something wasn't right. I sometimes became ill, and I felt that I had to go to the house of my godfather. When I arrived there I found my [objects of] Oyá kept apart from all other things. He did this in order to make me come there and spend money and do different works. I asked him about this, but he said it was nothing. Then I "asked" my stone of Oyá. I washed the stone in a herbal mixture. I had a "mental communication" with the stone. Words came to me in my mind, and the stone "told me" to visit a high priest, babalao. My godfather didn't like the idea, but I went there anyway.
>
> The babalao divined, and he said, "[The divinity and lord of divination] Orula is speaking here saying that you are preparing to do santo." I said, "Yes, I have everything prepared. All the animals and the clothes." He told me, "If you make that santo, you will not come out alive. You will die on the throne. Your santo is not Oyá, it's Obatalá. But to be more sure we have to find three more babalaos and use the *tablero* (divining tray), where Orula will speak directly to you."

The four priests divined and confirmed that the santo Eva had to make was Obatalá, not Oyá: "The medio asiento was well done, and Oyá helps me and defends me, but that was not the santo I had to make. When my godfather came to my house, he understood that he had done wrong and began to visit me less frequently. Then he became ill and had heart problems, and I haven't heard from him since." Eva also met others who tried to take advantage of her desperate situation. A palo monte priestess told her that she had to throw all her santería objects away and receive them again through her. On another occasion, a santera told Eva that the santo she had to make was not Obatalá but Oshún. Eva was confused, and her struggle against her illness went on.

The sense of coolness and of something supernatural in her body came back: "Sometimes I became very cold. I was shaking and my teeth were chattering. I also had a lot of pain in my head. My husband took me to the hospital. First they thought I had *nervios* [nervous problems], and then high blood pressure. But the blood pressure was normal. Later I understood that it was my guardian angel, Obatalá, who manifested its presence in this form. It wasn't blood pressure or anything, it was the santo. Obatalá was telling me that I had to make santo. When I made rogation of the head, the headache went away."

Eva heard about another santero who had helped many with serious health problems, and she went to his house for a consultation: "Everybody had told me different things. A lot of people had tried to use my situation and take my money, but this santero was different. He threw the [cowrie] shells and explained everything at once. He told me about my illness, that I had to do santo, and that it was Obatalá that I had to make. He told me secrets and problems about my life that only I knew about. I said, 'With him I will make santo.' I prepared everything very fast, and within two months I made santo. He became my new godfather." Eva did not know what would take place during the initiation. She was frightened and worried that she was doing something against her Catholic faith:

> My Catholic faith is the most important for me because that is the religion I have practiced since I was a child. I was worried that I was doing something wrong against God and Jesus. The first day of the initiation I prayed a lot to God. I was given food and I slept on the floor. When the ceremonies began, all my doubts disappeared, and I felt very calm. During the divination (itá), I was told not to eat sweet potato, egg, or intestines of any animal. I was also told that I could not travel in a boat or ride a train because there could be an accident where everybody would be saved, but I would die. The day after itá I made the presentation for the drums and danced in my beautiful white dress. I was like dizzy, it was very strange, very emotional.

During *el día del itá* (the day of divination), Eva was also advised about her religious faith: "They explained to me that I should not work with santería; my santos are only for myself. I was told about my relation to the church and that I should go to the church and pray when I have problems. I was also told to have nothing to do with sorcery. With sorcery you can do both good and bad, but here in Cuba it's mainly bad, and I don't like that. I was also told that espiritismo is very important in my life. The santos told me that I had to work a lot with espiritismo and help others to resolve their health problems."

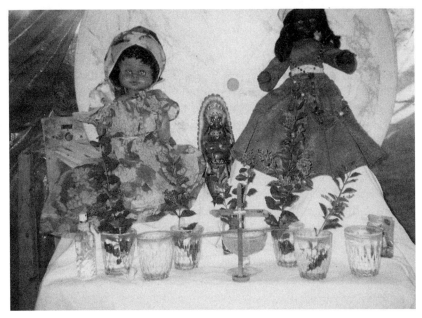

Fig. 3. Spiritist table. The dolls and the Plains Indian statue are personal spiritual protectors of the espiritista. Photo by Johan Wedel.

According to Eva, her illness has been a way for the santería divinities to tell her that she had to become initiated. "Otherwise I would not be in this religion, otherwise I would not be happy," she says. She also claims that she sees herself today more as an *espiritista* (spiritist) and Catholic person than as a santera. Spiritism is nothing new to her; she has felt the presence of spirits since she was a child.

Before Eva became initiated, she became involved in spiritism and made her own bóveda: "When I was seven I had my first religious experience. I went to the cemetery with my mother to put flowers on the grave of my grandfathers. When I came back I felt a strange cold in my body, and then a strange heat. I went to bed but it did not go away. An old lady cleansed me with an herb and told me not to go back to the cemetery, and I never did. Then, about a year later, I began to see things that were not natural. Once I saw a gypsy woman with a large skirt under a tree at the back of our house. I began to scream, and she disappeared."

When she became older, Eva had a dream that she today interprets as a spiritual message: "I saw my face in a window. The face changed to a round white face, and on the head there was a turban with a triangular stone in the middle. In the dream I knelt, and the image gave me a bunch of flowers and told me that I deserved it. Then, other images came with sticks and herbs from the forest and gave them to me." Today, spiritism is important in Eva's life, and she often helps people who have health problems:

> Spiritism has a very great power, and I have evidence of the power of spirits. I have been told to "develop" my spirits but have not done that, but they communicate with me. There is something mystical about my person that makes sick people better. They become healed. It's normal for me. A friend of our family, for example, had a serious problem with his knee, and he wanted to have an operation. One day he was here in the house in a lot of pain. I knew I could help this man. I lit a candle on the spiritist table and prayed to God, and I felt a strange force that was not normal. The man became better and has not had any problem since.
>
> The spirits tell me when someone is ill and what should be done. It comes to my mind that I have to do this or that. One day my husband had a very high fever and had to go to the hospital. It came to my mind that there was something supernatural about this. I went to my spiritist table, where I have four seashells, and asked [divined] if his illness had something to do with sorcery. The shells responded "yes," and I asked what to do. He had to be cleansed with smoke from a cigar and bathed with vencedor [a plant; literally, victor], pulverized eggshells, and perfume.

Both spiritism and santería have become important for Eva and have changed her life. Her recovery and ability to heal others has made her view her own life in a new way: "I was born to help people and I was born to become a santera. I made santo because of health problems. It's my way in life. When I entered into santería my health became much better. Every day I feel calmer. I feel more peaceful and secure, like someone is protecting me. My santos are my family, they are beside me and mean a lot to me. My godfather [the santería priest who performed the initiation] is also my new family. He means very much to me and is in my heart. I consider him my father, and I am his daughter. If I have a problem, he must help and protect me. I must also help him, it's my obligation. I trust him more than my own family."

Eva's Husband, Antonio

Eva's struggle against illness concerns not only herself but also the other members of her family. Eva's husband, Antonio, has been especially affected. He is Eva's third husband. In Cuba, it is common to marry three or four times during a lifetime, and Eva is no exception. Due to the difficult economic situation, many are under constant pressure to resolve basic problems such as acquiring food and other necessities. A married couple often has to share a small apartment or house with parents and other relatives, and arguments and fights may lead to discord and a divorce. Women also frequently divorce their husbands because the husbands are unfaithful over a long period of time. Eva and Antonio have lived together for about twenty years, and Eva's struggle against illness has also become her husband's:

> After my wife had her heart operation, I had to take her to the hospital at least once a week and spend the night there with her. They did an electrocardiogram and sometimes she had to stay a few days. She was in a very bad condition. I was usually away from work one day every week. I didn't know anything about santería at the time. When she said that she wanted to consult a santero, I told her that anything that could be beneficial for her health was okay with me. She has been my wife for a long time, and she is the mother of my child. I wanted her to become healthy and live her whole life.
>
> When Eva became involved in santería, she slowly became better. When she made santo she changed completely and her health became much better. Look at her now! She is drinking beer, she is very strong, she works very hard, she rises at four every morning and goes to bed late. After the operation, the doctors said that she couldn't even smell a beer or a soft drink. There were many things she couldn't eat or do. Today she lives like a normal person. It was not only her health that changed but also her personality. She's like a new person now. She is very tranquil and analyzes her problems. Before, she was a real headache. Twenty-four hours a day she was fighting. She argued with everybody and had terrible fights with her daughter who now lives in the United States.

Antonio claims that he used to be an atheist but that he has changed his mind after all his wife went through: "I never believed in any religion. But because of what has happened and what I have seen, I have come to the conclusion that something supernatural exists. Today, my wife's godfather sometimes consults with the [cowrie] shells for me. If he tells me to do a cleansing, a bath, or sacrifice an animal, I do it with a lot of faith and I resolve my problem. I do it because I am convinced that I will feel better and that it will be good for me."

Eva's Daughter Amelia

Eva's ten-year-old daughter Amelia is also becoming involved in santería. She agrees with her father that Eva has changed: "My mother told me that when she was a child, she saw things. She made santo because of health problems. Before, she lived in the hospital because she was always ill. Then she made santo and now she is in the religion. She is more tranquil today since she made santo. One day when I was ill and had flu, fever, asthma, and felt dizzy, my mother talked to Obatalá, and I was bathed with flowers, perfume, cascarilla, and *agua bendita* [holy water]. After that I felt better."

Máximo, Eva's Godfather

Máximo, the santero who initiated Eva, is about fifty years old. He is well known for his great knowledge of santería and has many godchildren both in Cuba and abroad. When Eva visited him for a consultation, he did not know her and had never seen her before: "Eva was very ill when she came to my house. I divined and [the combination] Eyeúnle Tonti Eyeúnle, eight-eight, came up. It was with *aro* [illness], and it came from heaven. The letra spoke about leaving the earth and going to heaven. But it also came up that she could be saved if she made santo. Obatalá would save her from illness and death. Eva left very content and with a lot of faith. The doctors said she had a serious heart problem. A vein was blocked and she had only a few months left to live. She said that she didn't believe in the doctors. Instead, she was sure that the santo would save her."

After the first encounter with Máximo, Eva had to do various works. She performed a spiritist mass and a rogation of the head, and she gave comida para la tierra. A mixture of herbs and plants related to the divinity Obatalá, such as almendra, almácigo, algodón, and granada, was also prepared. Eva drank the herbal mixture. She was also cleansed and bathed with it. According to Máximo, these works also helped her to acquire enough money to become initiated: "Two months after her first visit, Eva made santo. She made a female [aspect of the divinity] Obatalá, and her 'father' is Shangó. She began to feel better and better, and when she went back to the hospital, the doctors said she didn't have to come back again. It is now three months since she made santo, and she did everything with a lot of respect and was very correct. She doesn't have pain, she is fat, and the doctors don't find anything wrong with her."

The two women presented here tell similar stories; neither of them was satisfied with the biomedical treatment she had received. As they turned to santería, they began to relate their illness problems to social relations and to the spirit world. For both Matilda and Eva, santería has become part of a long struggle against illness, a struggle that has involved their husbands and children as well. They have experienced great changes in their lives, concerning both their health and their social relations. In order to stay healthy, they have become dependent on their relations to humans, spirits, and divinities. How can we make sense of Matilda's and Eva's seemingly strange responses to illness? Their beliefs and actions must first be related back in time, to a history that begins more than a century ago when hundreds of thousands of Africans were transported as slaves to Cuba.

Cuba and the Formation of Santería

From Africa to the New World

The relationship to Africa is commonly expressed in Cuba by proverbs like "The one who doesn't have something from Congo has it from Carabalí" or "And your grandmother, where is she?" meaning that everybody has a drop of African blood in their family as a consequence of the slave trade. Perhaps as many as a million or more African slaves were brought to Cuba, with the greatest number arriving in the last thirty years of the period before the slave trade was finally banned in 1868 (Brandon 1993:43; Castellanos and Castellanos 1988). Despite the ban, slavery was not completely abolished until 1886 (Vélez 2000:7).[1] West Africans who were forced from their native land brought with them elements of West African culture to Cuba.

A substantial number of the Africans who arrived in Cuba during the nineteenth century were Yoruba, from present-day southwestern Nigeria. As a result of internal wars and warfare with neighboring tribes, the Yoruba-speaking peoples were in a state of weakness and confusion. Their territories were under attack from both neighboring Dahomey and the Muslim Fulani in the north. This, in turn, coincided with a growing demand for slaves in the New World.

The Yoruba, known for their artistic traditions, were among the most urban of the African peoples, but they never built a common political state. What they had in common were a language and general religious ideas. The expression "Yoruba culture" is a somewhat recent invention. It was used for the first time during mid-nineteenth-century colonialism. "Yoruba" refers today to some twenty-five subgroups that speak the Yoruba language (Drewal 1992:12).

In many African religions, such as the orisha tradition of the Yoruba, there was a belief in the existence of a supreme God and a pantheon of subordinate divinities similar to the kind of folk Catholicism that was brought to the New World. In both of these traditions, people appealed directly to the divinities to resolve all kinds of problems: "The parallel orientations of the Catholic hagiology and the Yoruba pantheon toward resolution of practical problems gave direction to these paths of correspondence. In medieval Europe and later in colonial Latin America, Catholics adjured God, Jesus, Mary, and, above all, the saints to cure what ailed them" (Voeks 1997:60).[2]

In Cuba the Yoruba-speaking people and their descendants were called Lucumí. The origin of the name Lucumí is not known, but references are often made to a kingdom known as Ulkumi (Castellanos 1996; Ramos 1996). Most of the Yoruba slaves were sent to, and settled, in the western provinces of Havana and Matanzas, and it was in this part of Cuba that santería later developed and made its greatest impact.[3]

The Yoruba religion was preserved to a certain extent in the *cabildos*, societies for mutual aid, religious devotion, and entertainment that were established for both free blacks and slaves in urban areas. The cabildos originated in Spain, where religious associations were created to provide their members with financial support, health care, and religious celebrations (Sandoval 1995:83). In Cuba these associations became *naciones* (nations), groups of people classified according to ethnic belonging. People from the Yoruba subgroups, for example, became the Lucumí nation, and later some of these nations became cabildos.

The cabildos, used as bases for revolts several times during the nineteenth century (Howard 1998), were first organized along ethnic lines and were sponsored by the Roman Catholic Church under the direction of a diocesan priest. The priests apparently hoped that people would in time give up their African customs in favor of Christian beliefs. The leaders of the cabildos were referred to as kings and queens, and dancing and drumming took place in the cabildos on Catholic religious holidays. It is probable that the dancing, which remained African in style and may originally have been associated with rituals, at times turned into religious ceremonies. It was probably in the Lucumí cabildos that santería evolved (Brandon 1993:71ff). The religious beliefs of the Yoruba were transformed and influenced by Roman Catholicism.

During the last two decades of the nineteenth century, the cabildos began to change, and membership became open to non-Lucumís. At this time the government also began to restrict the activities of the cabildos. A license was required, and each cabildo had to have a Catholic name (Ortiz 1992:11). By this time it also became possible to become a Lucumí through initiation. Following the Catholic *compadrazgo* institution, members became *ahijados* (godchildren) of a certain priest (Brandon 1993:75). Some of these cabildos are still functioning, such as the cabildo Santa Teresa (founded in 1816), which is dedicated to the divinity Oyá, and cabildo San Juan Bautista, dedicated to Ogún, both in the city of Matanzas.

In today's Cuba people usually use the term santo when they talk about a specific orisha, and, with a few exceptions, both the Yoruba name (with a Cuban accent) and the Catholic name are used. Generally, santería followers also consider themselves to be Catholics. Despite this Catholic influence, the fact that orishas are called santos, and that it is common to be baptized before being initiated into santería, it would be wrong to call santería a form of religious syncretism. There is little evidence of Catholic elements when one looks deeper into aspects of the religion, such as the practice of the babalao, the high priest (Canizares 1993:46; see also Palmié 1995:82).

Many Yoruba were also sent as slaves to Brazil and the island Trinidad, where a similar process took place. In Brazil, Yoruba beliefs and Catholicism gave rise to the religious tradition *candomblé*, which is flourishing today in the state of Bahia. Followers of candomblé appeal to their *orixás* (divinities) in order to resolve both everyday issues and serious problems, such as a life crisis or an illness. According to Voeks (1997:70), its "medicine represents a cohesive medical system." Despite this, candomblé was suppressed until recently and is even today sometimes accused of representing irrational and superstitious beliefs.

At the end of the nineteenth century, medical services were scarce in Cuba. The former runaway slave Esteban Montejo, who has given a first-hand account of life in Cuba at the time of the abolishment of slavery, recalls the situation: "There were no powerful medicines in those days, and no doctors to be found anywhere. It was the nurses who were half witches who cured people with their homemade remedies. They often cured illnesses the doctors couldn't understand. . . . The secret is to trust the plants and herbs, which are the mother of medicine" (Montejo 1968:42).

When sick, the majority of the blacks and many whites from the Creole population relied on African healing knowledge and medicinal herbs and plants (Sandoval 1995:91). In Palmira outside Trinidad, for example, a building that housed a famous cabildo was constructed with money from a slaveowner who wanted to thank his former female slave for curing his sick daughter with herbs (Orozco and Bolívar 1998). Also, in the twentieth century, hospitals and pharmacies "functioned alongside Yoruba and Kongo healers and diviners, and stethoscopes, divining chains and magical mirrors could all be found among the diagnostic tools available to the Cuban people" (Marks 1987:228). Despite this important knowledge, people of African origin were regarded as a source of labor and not as bearers of culture, until the abolition of slavery (Bastide 1971:1). This, in turn, has also led to intolerance toward Afro-Cuban religions. Periodically, throughout the nineteenth century in Cuba, ritual drums were prohibited and sacred objects were burned (Martínez Furé 1979:185).

In the last decades of the nineteenth century, relations between the government and the cabildos became increasingly strained as meetings and organizations of cabildos became restricted. During a campaign of nationalism and Europeanization, from 1902 through the late 1920s, the cabildos were subjected to persecution and confiscation of religious paraphernalia (Brandon 1993:82ff).

It was not only in the cabildos that people suffered from intolerance. In an interesting source of information about the practice of santería, its ways of healing, and its relation to the state in the beginning of the twentieth century, Ortiz presents extracts from the daily press in Cuba (Ortiz 1995:151ff). It should be noted that all kinds of magical practices are called *brujería* (sorcery) in the newspapers and that santería is not distinguished from the other important African-derived religious practice, palo monte. In 1903, for example, in Guanajay, Pinar del Rio, a group of about sixty people carried out a *celebración del santo* (celebration of the saint). In Macagua the Rural Guard surprised seventeen Afro-Cubans who were practicing acts of sorcery. Various objects were found, and a rooster was seen placed next to an altar. The judge condemned the group to twenty-five days in prison. In 1904, in a house in Havana, the police found two altars with images of two Virgins surrounded by feathers, coconuts, and candlesticks. In a corner were found a washbowl with blood, shells, a candle, and other objects.

From Güira de Melena it is reported that despite this "rich and apparently cultivated area" there are a lot of objects belonging to sorcerers thrown on the streets and on hedges. Similarly, in Havana, in a street named Picota, one could see objects of sorcery such as maize, feathers, and other "dirty objects." The newspaper finally urged the police chief in the area to put an end to this "bad" practice. Another newspaper in Cienfuegos reported, "There are neighborhoods in the city where only sorcerers live." The following year the police entered a house in Havana and found more than a hundred people practicing sorcery. A doll named Shangó, white and black stones, horns, dry coconuts, a skeleton of a goat, and other objects were found. Thirty-two women and twelve men were arrested. Some had been wearing masks, which may refer to the powerful santo Olokun who uses a mask to cover her face, although today Olokun does not possess devotees. According to Barnet (1983:186), this santo can only be seen in dreams, wearing a mask; those who see the face of Olokun will immediately die.

Knowledge of medicinal herbs and plants and healing have played an important role in the formation of santería. This role of santería as a means to heal ailments has a long history; during the nineteenth century, medical treatment was partly administered by healers of African origin and their pharmacopoeias. The cabildos, "as mutual help societies," also provided help to members in cases of illness and death (Brandon 1993:70ff).

The ex-slave Montejo stated, "No one had any faith in the Spanish doctors. It was still witchcraft which cured people" (Montejo 1968:93). He continued: "A Congolese or Lucumi Negro knew more medicine than most doctors . . . They could even tell when a person was about to die" (166). Different kinds of healing were often lumped together as "sorcery"; practitioners of these activities were also subjected to oppression and intolerance.

For example, in 1903, in the street of San Joaquín, Havana, a man was arrested for having dedicated himself to healing with herbs and beverages and for possessing numerous objects used for sorcery. He claimed that he cured people, following his ancestors who were Lucumí, Gangá, and Arará (Ortiz 1995:153). In the village of Cabezas, a man is said to have carried out various cures with herbs. From Batabanó and Colón there are also reports of sorcerers working as healers (166ff). The following year, in a house in the village of Managua, there was a report of people dancing "el Santo," carrying out sorcery sessions, and healing. Cockerels, ducks, and pigeons had been sacrificed to heal some children. A doll called Santa Bárbara, shells, herbs, beverages, and other items were found in the house.

Intolerance of the Afro-Cuban religions continued well into the 1920s and 1930s, although the artistic movement of Afro-Cubanism, *afrocubanismo,* with its interest in African and Afro-Cuban culture, made it possible to view and present santería "as folklore rather than witchcraft and crime" (Brandon 1993:93). Painters such as Wilfredo Lam and writers such as Alejo Carpentier and Nicolás Guillén made Afro-Cuban culture known to the world. Nevertheless, Afro-Cuban religions continued to have a negative public image in the 1940s.

Santería after the 1959 Revolution

Santería was, to a large extent, practiced in secrecy during the first two decades after the Cuban revolution in 1959, and "relations between religious groups and the socialist state oscillated between tolerance and repression" (Brandon 1993:100). During the 1960s in Cuba, the new socialist government treated the Afro-Cuban religions with suspicion and hostility, and "restrictions were placed on their functioning; their leaders were often arrested and sometimes imprisoned; their adherents encountered discrimination in employment" (Segal 1995:236).

Devotees were accused of involvement in antirevolutionary activities, and their meetings were banned or subjected to approval (Barnet 1988). Religious affiliation could impede advancement in the workplace (Rabkin 1991:189), but this discrimination was less harsh than that experienced by followers of Catholicism and Protestantism. Since there is no centralized hierarchy and leadership in santería, the government probably found it less threatening to the ideas of the revolution.

The National Institute of Ethnology and Folklore was founded in 1961. The establishment of the institute had to do not only with scientific interest; the government also wanted to better control the Afro-Cuban religions, partly because they constituted an informal economic network that did not fall under the control of the centrally planned economy of the state.

During the 1970s, relations between the government and Afro-Cuban religions relaxed slightly. In 1976, the freedom to profess any religious belief was guaranteed in the Constitution. During this period, Cuba also became more militarily involved in Africa, and interest in the continent increased. In a well-known speech on December 22, 1975, at the Plaza de la Revolución in Havana, Fidel Castro declared that "we are not only a Latin American country, but also an Afro-Latin country. . . . The blood of Africa runs abundant in our veins."

Despite this, restrictions continued and participation in santería was not openly displayed in the 1970s. Permits for ceremonies that included drumming were difficult to obtain, and minors were not allowed to become initiated. People who were active in the Communist Party were prohibited from practicing the religion. This was expressed in a study by Oscar Lewis and his team by a fifteen-year-old girl when discussing a friend: "I'm pretty sure he isn't a *santero* because he belongs to the Youth and they'd kick him out in a minute if he got mixed up with such things" (Lewis et al. 1978:510).

At the end of the 1970s, the government began to promote secular versions of Afro-Cuban religions, presenting them as folklore rather than religion. The Cuban National Folklore Ensemble was created. At the same time, religious practice was said to be irrational and primitive. Practitioners were accused of antisocial tendencies and low moral values. Santería's tolerance toward homosexuals and people with alternative lifestyles was seen as a threat to society.

The situation gradually changed during the mid-1980s. Private farmers' markets were permitted as Cuba began opening up toward the outside world by inviting foreign investment companies and by building up a tourist industry. In this climate, religious practice in general became better tolerated. Relations between the government and the Roman Catholic Church were relaxed. This coincided with the publishing of a book in which Fidel Castro was interviewed about his religious life (Castro 1987). Many santería devotees I met claim that the more easygoing attitude of the government toward santería was a result of the book's publication.

Another important sign of a changing attitude and of reconciliation was the official visit of the spiritual leader of the Nigerian Yoruba, the Ooni of Ifé, Alaiyeluwa Oba Okunade Sijuwade Olubuse II, in 1986. Ooni met with high-ranking officials of the Politburo, including the head of the Ministry of Culture, Armando Hart Dávalos, and President Fidel Castro. The meeting was arranged by the head of the Office of Religious Affairs, Afro-Cuban specialist José Carneado Rodrígues. He had previously visited santería ceremonies and arranged meetings with babalao priests and officials of the regime.

During the 1980s, many African students were educated in Cuba, and exchanges on different levels took place with several African nations. Articles about Afro-Cuban traditions became more frequent in Cuban newspapers and journals. Some babalaos created the first institutionalized group of priests, called Ifá Yesterday, Ifá Today, Ifá Tomorrow (*Granma International* 1988; Vélez 2000:92f). This organization was later followed by another constellation, the Asociación Cultural Yoruba (Yoruba Cultural Association), which many babalaos joined.

Beginning in the early 1990s, religious believers were permitted to join the Communist Party, and Cuba was declared a secular rather than atheist state. In 1992, the Fourth International Congress of Orisha Tradition and Culture took place in Havana. The congress was arranged by the Yoruba Cultural Association, and delegates from Nigeria, Benin, the United States, and Puerto Rico met with Cuban santería priests, researchers, and dignitaries in discussions, seminars, and visits to Afro-Cuban museums.

The visit of Pope John Paul II in 1998 represented a further step toward relaxation of the relationship between religious practitioners and the state.

The pope met with Catholic, Protestant, and Jewish religious leaders. The babalaos, represented by the Asociación Cultural Yoruba, also wanted to meet with the pope. Unfortunately, their request was turned down by the authorities of the Roman Catholic Church in Cuba. This came as a great disappointment to the babalaos and all santería practitioners, who felt themselves marginalized by the whole ecumenical community. For many santeros and babalaos, the decision was evidence of the conservative and inflexible stance of the church.

Some churches in Cuba, such as the Pentecostal Church, call Afro-Cuban religions the work of the Christian devil. The Protestant and Roman Catholic Churches on the other hand, take a less harsh position although they also have a negative attitude toward santería and related traditions. A friend of mine, for example, who was studying at the Cuban Episcopal Church, conducted a study of santería. He wanted to present his work to the other students but was not allowed to do so. The reason given was that the students should not engage in obscurantism.

Afro-Cuban religions have traditionally been regarded as obscurantism by the Roman Catholic Church, but as most santería followers also consider themselves Catholic and frequently visit the churches, some priests have tried to show a positive attitude toward santería. Holding the view that it is easier to convert souls among believers than among atheists, some priests in neighborhoods with a strong Afro-Cuban tradition turn a blind eye to santería activities inside and outside the church. Such an attitude is not, however, approved of by the church authorities.

During the 1990s, santería was practiced more openly. It is now visible everywhere in Cuba, and people of all ages are becoming initiated. As one santera said, "Today we can wear our necklaces without fear." According to a maker of sacred santería drums: "There was a witch-hunt against the religions here and now it's just the opposite. Everyone's religious. Now everyone wears a bead necklace" (Benkomo 2000:143). The change is partly due to a more relaxed attitude from the Cuban government; partly due to the fact that people see santería healing as a powerful alternative and complement to biomedicine; and partly because the economic crisis has given belief in santería new force, as people use the tradition to resolve problems related to the crisis.

Santería today attracts tourists and other foreigners. The tourists, who come to Cuba from all over the Americas and Europe, are usually interested in the folklore. They may occasionally attend rituals and divination sessions in private houses. Other foreigners become personally involved in rituals. Many of these are Cuban exiles and people from neighboring countries.

Often, their main reason for coming to Cuba is initiation because of an illness. In a santero's house in Matanzas, for example, I met a Mexican woman who was waiting for a divination session. She had lung cancer and had recently visited the nearby hospital. With her X-ray plates in her hand, she was now waiting to hear what the santero had to say about her problem.

Some of these visitors learn how rituals are performed and then initiate others in their home country. Both groups bring highly-sought-after hard currency to the country, which is probably an important reason for the relaxed attitude from the government toward the Afro-Cuban religions.

Another possible reason is that these traditions are so popular that it would be useless to try to hinder their practice. The secretary-general of Cuba's Catholic episcopate, Monsignor Carlos Manuel de Céspedes, estimated that about 85 percent of the Cuban population of about eleven million practices some form of Afro-Cuban religion today (Moore 1988:344). Santería is the largest one, and its followers can be found all over Cuba, although the majority live in the western provinces of Havana and Matanzas (see Argüelles Mederos and Hodge Limonta 1991).

Santería today attracts people from all strata of Cuban society. Initiates can be seen everywhere in their white clothes, but most followers are Afro-Cubans. The religion has traditionally been strong among people of African descent and is more common in working-class, low-income neighborhoods dominated by Afro-Cubans, such as Jésus María y Belén in Old Havana, and Simpson or La Marina in Matanzas.

The Cuban government uses popular culture and artistic expressions to achieve the goals of the revolution, to support the socialist ideology (Daniel 1995:143), and to profit from the rapidly growing tourist industry. As the Afro-Cuban traditions move out into the public sphere, they become more commercialized. Openness toward these traditions has also brought a wave of artistic expressions and Afro-Cuban painting, dance, music, and theater, and these are steadily gaining importance in Cuban society. The well-known naïf paintings of Afro-Cuban myths by Cuba's most important painter, Manuel Mendive, represent one example.

In the small street Callejon de Hamell in central Havana, there is another interesting example of recent Afro-Cuban artistic expression. The artist Salvador Gonzalez has painted the walls with Afro-Cuban motifs. Here, rumba music, which may contain santería songs and movements, and dance and quasi-religious ceremonies attract both tourists and locals. In 1996, for example, a *vodou* dance was performed, accompanied by the sacrifice of a goat (a form of Haitian vodou is practiced in Cuba today, mainly in the province of Camagüey).

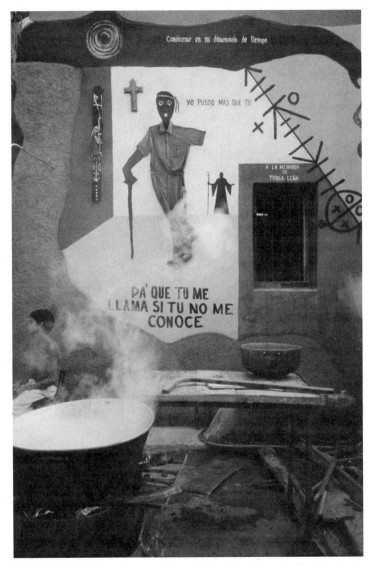

Fig. 4. Afro-Cuban objects and motives in the small street Callejon de Hamell in Havana. The text on the wall reads: "Why do you call me if you don't know me." The phrase is often used in spiritism sessions when spirits are called upon. Photo by Johan Wedel.

Santería is also present in many salsa songs and other kinds of popular music. A famous music group is called Los Orishas, and the singer Celina recently had a hit with the song "Que viva Chango." Other examples of the conscious exhibition of Afro-Cuban cultural elements include a popular liquor called "Santero," marketed as "the liquor that opens the roads," and a state-owned machete factory a few years ago named Ogún. Numerous popular books about Afro-Cuban religions have also been published in Cuba in the 1990s and can be found in many bookstores.

Outside Cuba, information and stories about santería are also spreading rapidly through publication of santería manuals and popular books. In many of the more popular publications, which are brought to Cuba by visitors, it is common to find amazing stories about how people have been healed or become ill through santería.

After the revolution many Cubans left for the United States, where santería is now growing fast among both Hispanic and non-Hispanic communities. Most practitioners are to be found in Miami and New York, although the religion is now widespread in the country (Canizares 1994; Curry 1997:10). Santería ritual specialists travel all over the country to perform rituals, creating links between distant groups (Brandon 2002).

In the United States, the networks and social support acquired through santería have been important for many Cuban exiles in resolving socioeconomic problems and other stressful experiences by giving a sense of belonging (Sandoval 1995:94; Gregory 1987). Based on a study in Dade County, Florida, Sandoval argues that santería "now constitutes a sprawling, vital and dynamic mental health care system" (1979:137). According to Sandoval, many of these immigrants suffer from feelings of powerlessness and a confused identity, and seek santería treatment (see also Jones et al. 2001; and Pasquali 1986, 1994).

Santería is also practiced today in most Latin American countries and in Europe. Although there are fewer Cubans living in Europe, there is a growing interest there in santería. In Göteborg, Sweden, for example, I recently met a Cuban babalao who performed divination for clients who frequently consulted him because of health problems. I also encountered a Mexicanborn santera who had been initiated in Havana and who was about to begin initiating others.

Santería, Health Care, and the Economic Crisis

Since the 1959 revolution, health care has been considered to be both the right of the people and a state responsibility. In the 1960s, priority was put on provision of care for patients suffering from acute infections, development of a network of health services, and training of health personnel. During the 1970s and 1980s, mortality and morbidity rates fell in tandem with an increase in life expectancy. Preventive care was prioritized. Between 1958 and 1988, life expectancy rose from 57 to 74 years, while the infant mortality rate (per thousand live births) decreased from 60 to 13.3 (Stubbs 1989:v). In 2000, the infant mortality rate for children under the age of five had decreased further, to 9 (UNICEF 2002).

There have been major investments in biotechnology, health tourism, foreign medical student programs, medical conferences, and international medical aid programs through which Cuban physicians have been sent to Third World countries as aid workers. This has given Cuba much political prestige both at home and abroad. According to Feinsilver (1993:200), the government puts high priority on health in order to achieve legitimacy, and Fidel Castro "is thought by many to be the real minister of health."

In 1985, a "family doctor" program was gradually introduced, which further increased health services. In the program, physicians live and work in a neighborhood with six to seven hundred people, and health and socioeconomic information is collected for every person (Stubbs 1989:94f). The family doctor clinics and the emphasis on preventive care enhanced the government's legitimacy, but the high ratio of physicians to population also made Cuba an "overmedicalized society" (Feinsilver 1993:199). Cuba's health care services began to change with the downfall of Communism in Eastern Europe. Until 1990, though, according to Feinsilver, "The revolution provided a sense of security, a freedom from fear of illness . . . because people knew that if they became ill, they would be given the best possible care without prejudice or charge" (202).

Cuba was severely affected by the collapse of the Communist regimes in Eastern Europe because the Soviet bloc accounted for a large part of Cuba's trade. An economic crisis, the so-called special period, began in 1990. Fuel became scarce, many factories had to close down, and public transportation almost came to a halt. This, in turn, led to diminishing food rations, scarcity of consumer goods, and frequent power outages that sometimes lasted for many hours.

Within a few years, the economy fell by about 50 percent. The crisis persists at the time of writing. The economy has recovered slightly since the worst years of 1993 and 1994, but few have seen any improvement in their living conditions. The special period is still very much a reality for those who lack access to U.S. dollars.

Most people are suffering and struggling to fulfill their most basic requirements, and this is reflected in responses to the common greeting

"How are you?": *Aquí, en la lucha* ("Here, in the struggle"), or *No es fácil* ("It's not easy"). Some have likened Cuba to a *palenque*, a settlement for runaway slaves (Pérez Sarduy and Stubbs 2000:6). The changes that struck the Cuban population were described by one writer in the *New York Review of Books* as "an event as inconceivable and shattering as the arrival of the Spaniards on Mexico's shores was for the Aztecs" (Guillermoprieto 1998:22).

Felicia is thirty years old and lives in Havana. She remembers how everything around her changed:

Before the special period we were quite happy. We got most food and clothes on the ration book at a very low price. There was plenty, and the things that were not on the ration book, like conserves and biscuits, could be bought at a low price in the shops. When the special period arrived, things changed slowly at first. We noticed that there were fewer things on the ration book for each person. After a few months clothes, shoes, meat, cooking oil, soap, and washing powder almost disappeared. There was nothing to buy in the shops, either. We still received small quantities of rice, beans, sugar, eggs, and bread. Children and old, sick people also received some milk and meat.

First we bought rice and beans from the farmers, but as the prices rose we could not continue with that. Some people became very thin. There were power failures for sometimes twelve hours, and people had problems getting to work because there were few buses. It became difficult to get medicines. Many got problems with their nerves. I saw a lot of people who turned crazy and were talking to themselves on the street. Many, especially single mothers with children, tried to kill themselves with pills. Many tried to escape on rafts to the United States.

After awhile they opened shops with products from abroad with prices in dollars, but as our salaries were very low we could not buy anything. Then the tourists came and prostitution rose incredibly. Many with high education left their jobs to become prostitutes. There was a lot of envy between neighbors and people began to steal. There was much more violence. We got more police, and some of those who criticized what was happening were put in jail. I saw a great difference between those who had access to dollars and those who had not. That was when I understood that this was nothing temporary. It was going to continue. The situation is the same today; it is like two different worlds within the same country. All this struggling makes me very tired. I feel that sometimes they even take away the desire to live. Many of my friends don't want to have children because of this [situation].

Many I met had a similar story to tell, and people often expressed how insecure they felt by saying, "I don't know what is going to happen to me," or "I don't understand what is happening." Some claimed that they were almost starving while politicians, high-ranking military officers, and foreign tourists were living in luxury. "Everything is for them and there is nothing for us," they said. Many spent several hours every day trying to "resolve things." People were constantly discussing food, food prices, what they had been eating, what they were going to eat, or where they had acquired the food. Before the special period began people were accustomed to eating well.

Because of the food shortage they are now growing "thin" in the same way that the whole society is deteriorating. Becoming thin "does not only mean becoming less attractive, less womanly or manly but in a way also means being less Cuban. Being Cuban has for more than thirty years been related to the revolution. The revolution has 'given' people the opportunity of being real Cubans, real men, real women, by giving everyone access to food and a decent life. Losing this base leads to much confusion and makes it difficult for many to understand what the 'revolution' is today" (Rosendahl 1997b:160).

Some also claimed that the problem was ideological. A woman in her mid-fifties, who was an active member of the Communist Party in the 1970s, claimed that "the greatest mistake of the revolution was the failure to acknowledge that people are different from one another. The young people today want to be themselves, not some kind of collective robots."

"Pessimism, apathy, and cynicism have replaced revolutionary fervor" (Suchlicki 2000:57), and all sectors in society have been affected by the crisis. The situation was made worse by the tightening of the U.S. trade embargo in 1992 in the form of the Torricelli-Graham Act, extended in 1996 in the form of the Helms-Burton Act. The health sector was deeply hit, and the quality of health care was reduced because of the scarcity of drugs and medical supplies. According to the American Association for World Health (1998:130), the embargo has "dramatically harmed the health and nutrition of large numbers of ordinary Cuban citizens. . . . Since 1992 the number of unmet medical needs (patients going without essential drugs or doctors performing medical procedures without adequate equipment) has sharply accelerated."

Most people first go to the hospital or the family doctor in the neighborhood when someone gets ill or needs some sort of medical assistance. Health care is still free and well developed. In spite of this, people do not have the same confidence in hospital treatment as they had before the special period began. It is common that medical equipment in hospitals does

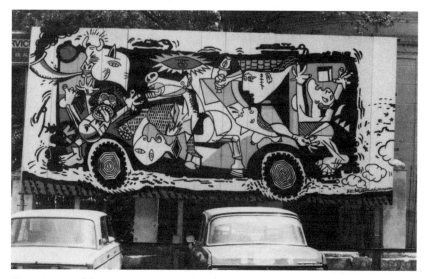

Fig. 5. Image of the crisis. In a travesty of Picasso's painting "Guernica," a view of the public transportation system is displayed. Photo by Johan Wedel.

not work or is missing. Sheets on the beds are lacking, water and electricity supplies are temporarily cut off, and medical personnel, also heavily affected by the crisis, are absent because they are somewhere else looking for food or some other basic necessity.

This is not to say that most medical employees do not work very hard. On the contrary, many have long working days due to poor public transport, and they struggle hard to give patients the best care available. Hospitals are sometimes referred to as *mata sanos* (killing the healthy), and there are many stories of people who went to the hospital for a minor problem and caught a severe disease or even died. Many carry out some kind of santería ritual before going to the hospital in order not to "leave in a worse condition than when entering." More than once I saw sacrificed fowls on the street outside a major hospital in Havana.

The Cuban state, which is responsible for all health institutions, previously guaranteed its citizens adequate treatment, and all kinds of chemical medicines were available at low costs. Today, with the economic crisis, many drugs on the market are only available in hard-currency pharmacies. There is also a lack of medicine in the hospitals. One answer to this lack of drugs has been to introduce herbs and plants on a large scale and to actively encourage the use of "green medicine." One of the side effects of this campaign has been that santería and palo monte are gaining recognition due to

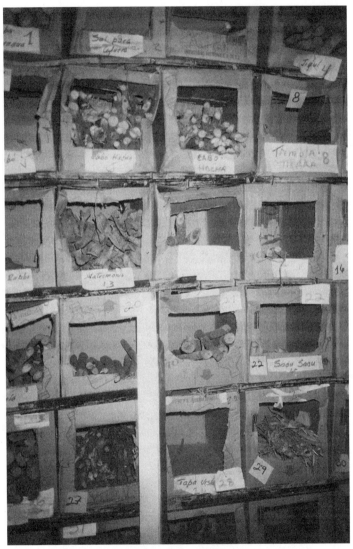

Fig. 6. Sticks and leaves for sale in an herbal store. On one of the boxes is written "Tiembla Tierra" (Shaking Earth), a name also given to a palo monte divinity. Photo by Johan Wedel.

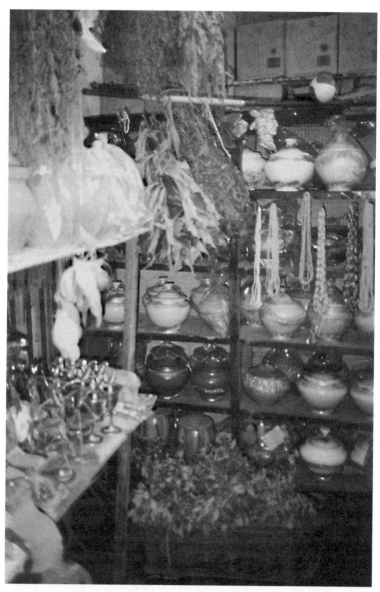

Fig. 7. Santería objects for sale at the yerbero. Photo by Johan Wedel.

their extensive knowledge of medicinal plants and herbs. These can be bought at the private store of the yerbero. In the store, which is often located in a room in a private house or in a garage, all kinds of herbs, plants, and religious paraphernalia are sold.

Information on the use of herbs and plants is being spread to the population and to medical personnel. Special pharmacies retailing only medicinal plants and herbs have opened. At one of these pharmacies in Matanzas, a sign proclaimed that herbal medicine had nothing to do with poverty. It was signed by Raúl Castro, minister of the Armed Forces and brother of Fidel Castro. A woman who is both a santera and palera explained: "There was a time when herbs were related to obscurantism and sorcery and you could not even mention it. But now it's the other way around. Now the first thing you need to know about is herbs, and they even give programs on the radio about the green medicine."

The medical properties of many plants and herbs have been known for a long time by part of the population and by botanists and folklorists. Cabrera (1993a) and Roig y Mesa (1988), for example, list hundreds of medical, aromatic, and poisonous plants and how they are used. But plants and herbs cannot replace all chemical drugs, and Cuban physicians often find themselves in a difficult situation. They prescribe herbal medicine knowing that the drugs they would like to prescribe are not to be found, or they might prescribe a chemical drug hoping that the patient can find it.

In most pharmacies where medicines are sold in local currency, the shelves are almost empty and herbal medicines often are offered instead of chemical drugs. People queue in vain with their prescriptions from the hospital or their family doctor; the common response in the pharmacy is "We don't have it." The lucky may find the drug after visits to four or five other pharmacies.

Often though, the drug cannot be found and the patient has to buy it either from a pharmacy that accepts only dollars, or use herbal medicine. The tragedy that follows when chemical drugs are not to be found has many faces. Outside a luxury hotel I met a mother with her baby in her arms, begging tourists for money so she could buy drugs for her sick child. On another occasion a neighbor came home crying because her twenty-five-year-old friend had died from an attack of asthma since there was no asthma medicine to be found. As a foreigner with access to dollars, I was often asked to buy urgently needed medicine in the dollar pharmacy that was impossible to find in the pesos pharmacy.

People in Cuba suffer from effects of the economic crisis in various ways. In the first years of the crisis, for instance, more than forty thousand people were affected by optic neuritis, an eye disorder caused by vitamin deficiency (Eckstein 1994:135). Many worry constantly about how to get food and other basic necessities for themselves and their families. Others are depressed and anxious. These feelings are commonly expressed by the term *nervios* (nerves), a broad folk syndrome of distress or emotional stress often originating in domestic or work relations. The malady, which is often chronic, is common among poor people in Latin America (Scheper-Hughes 1992).

An understanding of depression and nervios requires an understanding of how the crisis and social change have generated stressful experiences. In Cuba, nervios is manifested as nervousness, anxiety, depression, confusion, trembling and sweaty hands, aggression, difficulty in sleeping, hair loss, a "jumping" stomach, and itching of the skin. A woman from Matanzas, about forty years old, explained: "There are many people who have not adapted [to the crisis], people who are used to eating better. Many have small children and they don't know how to find food for them, not today, not tomorrow, or after tomorrow. They become more irritable and agitated. That's how problems with nervios begin."

In this situation santería and the healing powers of San Lazaro and other santos have become important for many people who have health problems related to the crisis, but it is important to point out that even if health issues are the most common reason for consulting a santería priest, there are other motives as well. People often seek help from santería and the related religious traditions of espiritismo and palo monte to deal with problems relating to matters such as state bureaucracy and emigration, or to get a job that is paid in dollars. A santería priest visited by many people wanting help with emigration jokingly complained that "people think this is an embassy."

Many who experience uncertainty and an insecure life situation and feel that they cannot control their own life have turned to santería to become empowered and spiritually protected. I often met people who said that santería gave them more strength in their struggle against the consequences of the crisis. A santería priest told me that it was easier for him to put up with the crisis because he was spiritually protected and received advice from the santos, which helped him to live a more tolerable life. The santos warned him through divination, in dreams, and during possession about impending problems such as illnesses and other dangers.

In sum, santería's adaptability and ability to respond to extreme situations, from the brutal and harsh conditions of slavery to the anxiety and lack of medicines during the economic crisis, have been vital for its survival and development. Today santería is flourishing, both in Cuba and abroad.

3

रेरेरेरे

Etiology and Healing

For the santería practitioner, the world is ruled by divine forces. Illness is prevented and healing is achieved by creating and maintaining relations with these divine beings and spirits. In this chapter I examine how humans interact with the otherworld, how they benefit from it, and how it may affect their lives. I discuss assumed causes of illness in relation to santería cosmology and spiritism, and ask what takes place when illness is understood in terms of sorcery. Finally, I inquire into the santería response to illness expressed through rituals, the reshaping of social relations, and the use of herbs and plants.

Illness and Its Causes

Santería relates sickness (aro or *ano*) to a larger whole, to a world of divinities and spirits, and to a person's social situation. Ill health may manifest itself as a lack of ashé, which, in turn, is related to an imbalance between "hot" and "cool" liquids and objects. Santería priests who divine are often consulted by people with sickness problems, and the priest often concludes that the person lacks ashé. Through the letras the diviner reveals the underlying cause of the illness and gives advice about what measures should be taken. Through each of the sixteen divination signs in the *dilogún* divination system, the santos "speak." In the case of illness, the relation between a specific santo and a letra will help the diviner to "diagnose" the problem because each santo, in turn, is related to certain illnesses and body parts. The diviner will also ask through further divination about the origin of the illness.

Divination may reveal that a certain illness is caused by a spirit of the dead who must be "developed" in spiritist sessions. The spirit may want the ill person to become an espiritista and work as a healer in the religious tradition espiritismo. The source of the illness may also be an evil spirit sent by an enemy through palo monte, and the client must engage in rituals to remove the spirit. A santero from Matanzas gave the following explanation of the divination process to Rodríguez Reyes (2000:75):

> When aro [sickness] comes up, you investigate which *camino* [way] it comes from. The camino can be *aro otonowa,* sickness that comes from the sky. It is the same as *aro elese Olodumare,* sickness from the hands of God. When this letra comes up, the person is sent to the doctor because it is he who is authorized to cure the person. He will also be told to do some "works" designated by the santo or the muerto [spirit]. When a sickness is produced by a muerto that is not getting enough attention, it is called *aro elese eggun.* It may also be a muerto oscuro [dark spirit] that someone has sent and that is causing sickness. All this must be asked.
>
> The sickness is called *aro elese ocha* when a person has a debt to the santo that he has not repaid or does not know about. This also happens to a person whose head is claimed by the santo, but the person does not fulfill [his obligation to become initiated]. Since the person is obstinate, the santo pinches him. *Aro elese Eledá* means that the person is sick because of his own head, because of disobedience. The person knows that he is doing something bad, but does it anyway. (italics added)

In order to get an idea of the most common reasons for consulting a santería priest and how conclusions from divination are drawn, I examined one hundred santería consultations. Together with a famous santero from Matanzas, I analyzed the results of his most recent divinations. He maintained a record of the people he had advised and was able to recall their reasons for consultation, the cause of the problem, and what he recommended. Among those he advised, some were visiting him for the second or third time, and a few were also santería initiates (see app. 2).

Illness proved to be the most important reason for consulting the priest. Of the one hundred persons, more than half came because of illness. The second most important reason for performing the consultation was family problems, followed by problems with the law. Half of the cases were said to be caused by sorcery. Only three were classified as "punishment" by a santo. Of those consulting the santero because of illness, about half were said to have problems related to sorcery.

In almost all of the cases, the priest recommended spiritual cleansing and/or a bath. In more than half of the cases, the consultant was advised to perform some kind of offering or sacrifice, to receive a necklace and/or Eleggua and the warriors, and/or to visit a medical doctor. In almost half of the cases the santero recommended initiation, to "make santo." Interestingly, in seventeen cases the person was advised to visit a doctor despite the fact that the reason for consulting the priest had been something other than illness.

Only small gender differences were evident. A slightly greater number of women than men were advised to "make santo." The only significant difference we found was when problems with the law were given as the reason for consulting the priest; eleven were men, but only three were women. In sum, the sample showed that illness was the single most common reason for consulting a santero, both among women and men, and that people who suffered from illness were almost always sent to the biomedical doctor. Some kind of spiritual "work," or ritual, was also recommended in almost all of the cases. The examination further showed that initiation was frequently recommended and that problems were commonly related to sorcery.

Although rare, divine punishment is often discussed and is frequent in narratives about santería. Punishment can take place when someone is disrespectful or offends the santos, as in the following story from Matanzas where a young man was punished for behaving badly toward other people who had close relationships to the santos. The narrative makes explicit the relationship between the divinities of the santería pantheon, represented through natural forces and human characteristics, and the fate and behavior of humans:

A twenty-five-year-old man was very violent and wicked. He mistreated his many girlfriends, his old mother, who was a "child" of Yemayá, and his father who was a "child" of Ogún. On one occasion he killed an old woman by beating her on the head with a domino table. She was a "child" of Oshún, and her sister cursed the man, evoking Oshún. The wicked man's mother became so exhausted by grief and fatigue when this happened that she said: "Yemayá, for how long am I going to support this?" Sometime later the young man left a party and crossed the old railway bridge in the center of Matanzas where the river runs out into the open sea. He slipped, fell into the river, and died. The funeral was attended by many santeros, and one of them became possessed by Shangó, who said to the mother: "Wasn't this what you asked for?"

For all santería devotees, it was obvious that the troublemaker had paid the price for his behavior. Yemayá, the owner of the sea; Oshún, the owner of the river; and Ogún, the owner of iron, who is said to live on the railway line, had punished the man, all at the same time. Hence, the santos can heal, but they can also cause illness, suffering, and death when enraged. In another case that was interpreted as divine punishment, a man in his early thirties had been told that he was born to become a high priest, babalao. He went through the first ritual step, called *mano de Orula,* but he left it there and almost forgot about the santos. One day he got a thrombosis in his brain and part of his body became paralyzed. Julio, a friend of mine and a babalao, explained:

This man was born to become a babalao, but after he "received" mano de Orula he didn't care much about it. He is a butcher, which is something powerful here, but he began to drink and do other stupid things. So the santo gave him a pinch and he had a thrombosis. Part of his body was as though dead, and he forgot things. Orula said [through divination] that he would be saved but that he had to make santo and thereafter become a babalao. His road [in life] was to help humanity. Orula also told him that he should continue with the treatment at the hospital but that it was not the [medical] doctors who would save him. It was the "sorcery doctor," *el médico brujo* [that is, the santero or babalao]. He promised to make santo and later become a babalao and carried out some *limpiezas* [ritual cleansings]. After five months he began to recover.

Another man was punished with an illness for not being active in the worship of his santos. He was disrespectful and had to pay a severe price for his offense. The man, who had been initiated a few years earlier, joined a Protestant church group. The group did not accept worship of the santos and related it to the Christian devil. Hence, the santero hid everything related to santería under his bed. One day he became possessed with his santo, Shangó, who was very angry. Shangó said that his "horse" would be punished. Three days later the man woke up half-paralyzed. He was told by Shangó that he had to carry out a drum ceremony for the santo, which was done a few days later. He became slightly better but still suffered from the paralysis.

These three examples show that the santos may also be perceived as the reason for an illness. The divinity wants either to punish the person for some wrongdoing or to "wake him up" and change his life. An alcoholic may, for example, get a serious illness in order to stop his drinking and change his life through initiation. To become initiated is then the only way of becoming well, and when health is achieved, the healing process is interpreted as a test or as evidence of the santos's great healing power.

Another reason for illness, and one which is often related to the economic crisis, is nervios (nerves) (see ch. 2). When someone feels depressed and confused and suffers from nervios, the head is said to be "hot" and might be cooled, refreshed, and balanced in the ritual called rogación de cabeza. During the ceremony, the santería priest repeats in Lucumí: "Release us from all bad things, from death, from crime, from illness, from shame." Since the color white is related to purity, coolness, and freshness (and to the santería divinity and lord of purity, Obatalá), only white objects and liquids are used.

The ceremony is also carried out for other reasons, for example, in order to prepare for other rituals (Brandon 1991:63). In a rogation that I myself went through (divination had revealed that I needed to calm down), a paste made of milk, white bread, coconut meat, dried fish, dried meat from a kind of ferret, cacao butter, and cascarilla were put on different parts of my body together with cotton. The mixture put on my head was secured with a white handkerchief that I was to wear throughout the night. As sexual activity is prohibited in connection with all rituals, I was instructed not to have any kind of sexual contact during the night.

In the morning the mixture was placed in the forest, in this case under a tree. On other occasions, sacrifices may be placed at a crossroads where the divine messenger and trickster Eleggua, who opens and closes the roads in life, is said to reside. Accordingly, the crossroads represents the intersection between the phenomenal world of humans and the otherworld of divinities.

Spiritual baths are also a common treatment for those suffering from nervios. In a *baño de desenvolvimiento* (development bath), for example, the afflicted pours milk mixed with water over the body. As milk is white and related to Obatalá, lord of peace and tranquillity, the bath is performed in order to gain stability and peace in life. In another bath for problems with nervios, the herbs paraíso and muralla are ripped and mixed with blessed water from the church, water from the sea, and cascarilla. The mixture should be used seven times while the person calls Yemayá for help.

Troublesome Spirits and the Evil Eye

The religious tradition espiritismo is important when discussing santería healing. The history of spiritism in Cuba, with its belief that people can communicate directly with the dead, goes back to the second half of the nineteenth century. During this time Kardecism, a spiritual movement founded by Hippolyte Rivail, or Allan Kardec, as he called himself, reached Cuba after spreading through Europe and North America. A variant of Kardecism, espiritismo, developed and provided an alternative to Catholicism. The movement had a scientific orientation, carried an implicit criticism of institutionalized Christianity, and borrowed knowledge of herbalism, Native American healing practices, and African magical beliefs (Brandon 1993:86f).

During the 1880s, espiritismo became so popular in Cuba that it was said to be a "spiritual epidemic" in the eastern part of the island (Argüelles Mederos and Hodge Limonta 1991:177). Through espiritismo, people found that they could talk directly with a spirit through a medium. This practice of healing also had an effect on santería as santería priests began to accept the existence of dark, disturbing spirits. In espiritismo these spirits were important when explaining illness and suffering.

During individual consultations or the *misa espiritual* (spiritist mass), the spiritist becomes possessed with a personal spirit of the dead in order to heal and give advice to people attending the consultation or ceremony. The spirit usually speaks in a Cuban Creole language that can be difficult for outsiders to understand. The spirit may give warnings of a possible forthcoming illness or about others who may spiritually harm the person in question, frequently because of envy. Those who suffer from an illness can also be sent to a santería priest or to the hospital for a medical exam. Often, an illness is said to be caused by someone casting the evil eye *(mal de ojo)*. This usually has its origin in envy, but some people are also said to be born with this ability and may cause harm, especially to children, unintentionally. When someone is afflicted by the evil eye, the espiritista may pray to San Luis Beltrán while making a cross in the air with the plant albahaca.

A common form of spiritist mass, where the participants sit in front of the table while praying and singing to different kinds of spirits and saints, is called *espiritismo de mesa.*[1] During the mass, a deceased family member may also descend and possess one of his or her former relatives. On one of these occasions, I witnessed a deceased mother possess one of her sons. She was very sad and said that her daughter, who was also attending the ceremony, could die if she did not change her life. The daughter was very thin and smoked too much. It was recommended that she stop smoking, change her diet, and go and live with one of her sisters.

Today in Cuba one can find in the home of a spiritist a bóveda, a table covered with a white cloth. On top of it there are usually photographs of departed family members, a crucifix, dolls, and glasses of water. The dolls represent spiritual guides, and each glass represents a particular muerto, often a deceased family member.

The guides are frequently said to have an African or Haitian origin and, often, to have been slaves. They may also be Gypsies, Arabs, or Plains Indians and are generally believed to be good at healing illness. An espiritista whom I met in Matanzas, for example, had a muerto that was a male Sioux Indian. With the help of the spirit, the espiritista healed people with her hands. She claimed that her body became more masculine and "Indian looking" when she began working with the spirit, and since the Indian had died of thirst, she had to drink constantly and always carried water with her.

A person is considered to be born with the gift to be an espiritista in order to heal and help others, but the spirit first has to be developed in a spiritual mass with the help of other spiritists. Since people also frequently participate to develop their often troublesome spirits, the mass is referred to as *la escuelita* (the little school). When the spirit is "developed" and has "a lot of light," it can be controlled by its medium and called upon, as explained by an espiritista: "I didn't begin to develop my spirit until a few years ago. This began when he [her spirit] threw me out of the bed. My husband wanted to take me to a doctor but I went to a spiritist group to develop it. I know his name and that he's an African or Haitian. He's here to help and to show mercy to people."

Not all who develop their spirits become practicing spiritists, just as not all who become initiated into santería become practicing priests. The spirit may have to be developed and controlled because it is causing serious problems, often some kind of illness.

Sorcery

Brujería is the name that both laypeople and devotees often give to the religious tradition palo monte. Generally, the word brujería can also be used in santería when referring to more practical "works" *(trabajos)* such as mixing a powder or carrying out a minor sacrifice in order to "get something done." Further, the term brujería is not necessarily used in its negative, evil sense; it may also describe something powerful that can be used to fulfill wishes and resolve all kinds of problems.

Palo monte (also referred to as *palo monte mayombe* or *Regla Conga)* has its roots in the Congo. During the slave trade, many Africans were taken from the Congo region to Cuba, and their religious beliefs followed them. Palo monte is practiced all over the island but is particularly strong in the eastern provinces.

The slaves from the Congo were known as "Congoles" and were distinguished from the Lucumi by their religious practice. According to the former runaway slave Esteban Montejo, the "Congolese were more involved with witchcraft than the Lucumi, who had more to do with the saints and with God" (Montejo 1968:34). In Cuba, the beliefs of the Congoles developed into the palo monte religion. In the process, palo monte exchanged ideas with espiritismo and santería (Matibag 1996). Today, it is common that a person practices both santería and palo monte. However, because all kinds of popular rumors and horror stories about its activities are common, palo monte is not openly practiced.

The most important santería divinities have their counterparts in palo monte. Accordingly, Yemayá is called Baluandé, Shangó is Siete Rayos, Ogún is worshipped as Zarabanda, and so on. In palo monte these divinities are given less importance than in santería (Castellanos and Castellanos 1992). More important in palo monte is the *prenda* (Spanish: "treasure" or "jewel"), a large iron cauldron often kept hidden in the backyard. The prenda, sometimes referred to as *el brujo* (the sorcerer), is said to be alive. It protects, and is quick to carry out the wishes of its owner.

A palero explained the relationship between the prenda and its owner: "The prenda is a living thing, like an animal. It does not have any feelings, not even for its owner. That means that you have to be sure to dominate it and not let it dominate you. You have to speak in a hard way and say things like 'I will throw you into the sea.' Don't give it too much [sacrificial blood] too frequently. It will get used to it and then take you, the owner" (see also Palmié 2002).

Sticks from certain trees and many other secret objects are kept in the prenda, and usually also human bones. The spirit of a dead person is said to reside in the prenda, and it is regularly "fed" with sacrificial blood from male animals such as dogs, pigs, goats, and cockerels. The palero continued: "The prenda must have a dead creature inside, or it will not work. Without a brain the body won't work. The prenda must also have [sacrificial] blood because this nourishes it. Without blood, the prenda cannot walk or carry out any work."

When a new prenda is made, it is always "born" from a "mother" prenda. The palera or palero who has made a blood pact with the prenda communicates with and controls the spirit in order to carry out magical operations. To be powerful, the prenda must be kept away from menstruating women because menstrual blood makes the prenda weak. The prenda's thirst for blood may also be dangerous, causing a menstruating woman to lose much blood.

The prenda's power to both heal and harm was expressed by the former slave Montejo: "A *nganga* [prenda], or large pot, was placed in the centre of the patio. The powers were inside the pot: the saints. People started drumming and singing. They took offerings to the pot and asked for health for themselves and their brothers and peace among themselves . . . Inside the pot they put a plant called star-shake, together with corn straw to protect the men. When a master punished a slave, the others would collect a little earth and put it in the pot. With the help of this earth they could make the master fall sick or bring some harm upon his family" (Montejo 1968:26).

This kind of magic, and the fear it provoked, was probably one of the few powerful weapons that the slaves had against their owners. Montejo describes the prenda as very powerful. He "saw many things done with these pots, terrible things—people killed, trains derailed, houses set fire to" (Montejo 1968:135). If the owner of the prenda wanted to get rid of someone, dust from a path where this person had been walking was collected and put into the prenda. "That person's life would begin to ebb away, and at sunset he would be dying" (34).

Palo monte's close relationship to santería can be seen in santería consultations, where advice about palo monte may be given. Upon the outcome eleven-six in the dilogún divination system, for example, a client who is initiated into palo monte is advised to attend the iron cauldron where the palo monte spirit is said to reside. Palo monte priests, paleros, are skilled in all forms of magical practices that may be used for both good and evil purposes. They have a wide knowledge of herbs, plants, and different substances that can be used to heal and resolve problems, or to cause illness and other "bad things." Paleros know how to make magical powders that may be put into the coffee cup of an unsuspecting visitor, and I was often told to be careful about where I had a coffee. When these powders are used to cause harm, dried toad, human hair, or fish bones are common ingredients.

This ambiguity makes palo monte both highly valued and feared. It can be used to heal an illness or make someone powerful and rich, but it can also hurt someone who has, for example, become scandalously wealthy during the struggle of the economic crisis. In this sense, palo monte is like sorcery in general: It "is both a resource for the powerful and also a weapon for the weak against new inequalities" (Geschiere 1997:16).

Compared to santería, palo monte is more pragmatic, and people often consult a palera or palero when they want to see a rapid solution to their problem. The prenda, the iron cauldron, is important for magical operations; it will carry out the wishes of its owner. Two kinds of prendas are used. The Christian prenda, *prenda cristiana*, is baptized with holy water and used for well-being only. The Jewish prenda, *prenda judía*, on the other hand, is not baptized (hence its name) and is commonly used for *trabajos malignos*, evil, harmful work, such as causing illness and death.

Evil, harmful sorcery that causes illness is often said to have been carried out by palo monte priests who have a prenda judía. None of the paleros I met said they had a prenda judía, and I was told by them that to have an unbaptized cauldron was very uncommon these days. The santeros and espiritistas I met had a different opinion and told me that they had clients almost daily who had been the victims of sorcery carried out through palo monte. It is also commonly held that there has been a sharp rise in cases of sorcery since the economic crisis began.

Sometimes it is recommended that a person receive a prenda through santería divination. When a prenda judía is recommended, the intention is often to strengthen an evil, immoral person. Some of the paleros I met claimed that the distinction between good and bad prendas may not always be so clear. One palera told me that the prenda cristiana may, on rare occasions, also be used for evil purposes if the crucifix that is often placed over the prenda is removed.

In santería, illness is frequently explained in terms of sorcery and related to envy between family members, neighbors, or colleagues at work. A neighbor, relative, or colleague may be accused of having sent an illness through sorcery, and an afflicted person is often told to stay away from certain persons. Sometimes, he has to change his life and move to another place in order to become well. Illness, then, occurs in the social body and is socially experienced. The question of *how* a person became ill is followed by the afflicted person's wish to know *why*.

Such ideas, associated with witchcraft and sorcery in general, were discussed in depth in Evans-Pritchard's classic work on Zande witchcraft (1937). He showed how illness was made meaningful in terms of Zande culture and related to social relations. Evans-Pritchard also demonstrated how Zande used "this-worldly" phenomena to explain the immediate causes of illness and misfortune but turned to witchcraft and asked "why me?" in order to find an underlying cause that was both embedded in social relations and morally satisfying (Good 1994:11).

When a santería priest divines for a client and the outcome points at sorcery as a possible cause, there is, implicit in the question "why," also the question "who"—"who did it?" Certain persons may have carried out sorcery, and it is important that the priest identifies these people and their motives. The feelings and characters of the evildoers become important in order to know how to get rid of the affliction and protect the client from further problems. Divination brings certainty where there is uncertainty, and when sorcery is believed to be the cause of the problem, the focus is more on agents than on the victim. In parts of Africa where divination is performed, one can find similar procedures. Among the Nyole in eastern Uganda, for example, the characters and feelings of those agents who may have affected a person are examined more often than those of the suffering victim (Whyte 1997:80).

By interpreting the myths related to the divination outcome, the priest will know when someone is, or will become, the victim of sorcery. This can be exemplified by an interpretation of the following myth: "Shangó had two mistresses, Oshún and Oyá. One day Oshún told Shangó's legitimate wife Obba that if she wanted to bind her husband to her and make Shangó as passionate with her as he was with Oshún, Obba should cut off her ear and serve it in the soup to Shangó. This she did. When Shangó saw Obba with a bandage over one of her ears and learned what had happened, he became enraged. He swore that Obba would forever be his legitimate wife, but he would never make love to her again. Obba blamed herself and committed suicide."

A santero gave the following interpretation of the myth: "This story is about love affairs and about sorcery in order to 'bind' someone. Oshún wanted to be with Shangó and to throw out the other woman. I tell the man who is consulting to take care of his woman so that she will not bind him and 'have him under her feet' [dominate the man]. If it's a woman who is consulting, she must take care so her man won't bind her and have her under his feet. It's the same."

There are many different ways to bind someone, and they often include body fluids such as menstrual blood, sperm, sweat, and urine. In a santería manual, the following "work" to "bind" a woman was described: "Cinnamon powder, sugar, hair from all parts of the woman's body, shit from a sick hen, nails from the woman's left foot and hand, and sperm from the man, are mixed together. Make the woman drink the mixture, preferably in a cup of coffee."

Santería priests use divination to identify the person who performed sorcery on a client, but they seldom actually give the name. They will only say that it is a woman or a man and give some indication of what the person looks like, or give other clues allowing identification. Paleros and some espiritistas, on the other hand, often give the name and even tell where the person lives. Envy is often said to be the reason behind sorcery, and, as a santero said, "Sorcery can be eliminated, but the envy and the gossip cannot be removed; I would have to put out your eyes and cut off your tongue."

During a divination session that I myself underwent, the divining santero claimed that an ex-girlfriend had performed sorcery on me in Sweden and that she was trying to finish me off completely. He assured me that he could remove the sorcery performed but not the hatred and the envy.

Envy may also be a reason for spreading rumors of sorcery in order to hurt someone. According to the santero, "Some people spread rumors of sorcery and say that I, for example, have performed sorcery on you, even though I haven't done anything. Then, we will be enemies. You and the person who spread the rumors will be friends." Both santeros and paleros to some extent compete for clients, and envy between them can be a reason for sending an illness or some other "bad thing" upon others. Santeros possess knowledge of how to send bad things, but I was always assured that this almost never occurs; santería is not supposed to be used to cause harm to others, and I never met anyone who described santería as being harmful. Despite this, instructions to harm and dominate others can often be found in manuals on santería practice and may also be learned from other devotees.

In order to make someone ill, for example, part of the work includes writing the name of the person seven times on a yellow paper, mixing the paper with certain seeds and other ingredients, and putting it in a red cup while expressing what one wishes should happen to the person. I was told that to kill someone, one work includes stabbing a piece of meat seven times and, together with some other ingredients, offering it to Ogún. After this, a doll with the same skin color as the person, a paper with the person's name, and a knife are buried at the foot of a ceiba tree.

When an illness is sent through palo monte sorcery, someone related to the intended victim might catch the illness, particularly if the victim is well protected. In this view, the boundaries of the self are not considered to be limited strictly to the individual but also encompass other family members. Therefore, relatives of successful santeros also need some sort of sorcery protection. However, this does not mean that people unrelated to santería are safe. One informant told Lydia Cabrera nearly fifty years ago: "It is very dangerous to live here without a protective talisman. Ay! Cuba is full of sorcery" (Cabrera 1993a:20). The following story, involving spiritism, is a case in point.

A woman had been ill for a long time. She had pain in her belly and in one of her feet. She also had problems breathing normally. The doctors could never find out what was wrong with her, I was told. She participated in a spiritist mass, and the woman in charge of the mass became possessed by her muerto. This particular muerto was said to be of Haitian origin and very

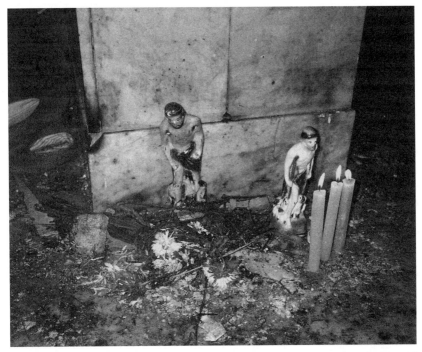

Fig. 8. Objects found inside the Church of San Lazaro. The flowers have been used for ritual cleansings against bad influences and sorcery. Photo by Johan Wedel.

good at healing. The spirit spoke through its medium to the sick woman about her work, her husband, her illness, and her life situation in general, and concluded that all her problems were due to sorcery. Another woman who was jealous of her success in life had sent a dark, evil spirit upon her.

Certain rituals were prescribed in order to take the evil spirit away, and a few days later the spiritist group met in a forest near Havana. The spiritist once again became possessed by her Haitian spirit, who cleansed the sick woman from the malignant spirit's power by passing a fowl over her body. She had been told to wear the same clothes for three days and nights and sweat a lot in them. The clothes were ripped to pieces and taken off. Finally, she was taken to the river, where her head was washed. Shortly after these rituals she felt better and, she says, has not had any problem since.

Two important ideas concerning sorcery are involved here: limpieza (cleansing) and rompimiento (breakage). In the three religious traditions mentioned in this work, limpieza is carried out with herbs and plants, fruits, an egg, a piece of meat, or a living fowl, any of which may be rubbed over the afflicted person's body. By this means, bad influences caused by other people's envy or sorcery are passed over to the object. When a fowl is used, it is later sacrificed but the meat is not eaten, as it is after most other rituals. An important limpieza is carried out with a chicken on the last day of each year so that the new year may be entered fresh, thus leaving behind all bad things caused by sorcery. Limpieza is not only carried out to ritually cleanse humans; cars and motorbikes can also be cleansed, usually with a bunch of leaves.

Ripping a person's clothes to pieces, rompimiento, is carried out in serious cases and usually through espiritismo and palo monte when a person must get rid of an evil spirit that may be troublesome. In santería this is often performed by making sacrifices to two orishas who are related to the dead, Oyá and Yewa. These cases are usually taken seriously since illness, madness, or even death is said to occur if nothing is done.

In the case of the Haitian muerto above, healing was similar to santería practice. The spiritist became possessed with a spirit that discussed the afflicted woman's life situation. The origin of the illness was related to her social world: an envious woman in her surroundings. By stating that an evil spirit was causing the problems, the illness was also given a name. This "naming" of the source of suffering can serve "to formulate the object of treatment and thus organize a set of social responses" (Good 1994:133). As discussed earlier, naming the source of the disorder is also common in santería, often by referring to the mythological events of the santos.

In today's Cuba, with the mounting struggle over hard currency and material goods, envy and sorcery are said to be common, which, in turn, may result in illness and misfortune. An envious person can cast a mal de ojo on another person. Small children are said to be especially vulnerable and therefore often use resguardos (protective talismans).

Envy is a common reason for acts of sorcery. People who in some way have succeeded in life are especially subject to sorcery. This is reflected in a recent song by the salsa singer El Médico de la Salsa, who, like most musicians, is very quick to pick up the latest trends in Cuban society and use them in a song: "Grandmother, what would happen if I, because of sorcery, slip and suddenly fall?"

When discussing clients' illnesses with santería priests, I was often told that the origin of illness lies in envy and sorcery. A common story was that a neighbor or someone in the family had carried out sorcery on the client because the person lived a better life or had managed to improve her or his situation. Many people I met during fieldwork were concerned with the individualistic and often egoistic view others were said to hold. As one man

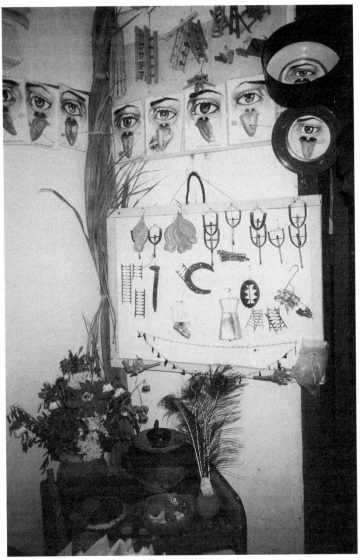

Fig. 9. Santería and antisorcery objects for sale at the yerbero. Photo by Johan Wedel.

said: "We live in a world with a lot of egoism, a lot of envy. Life is a competition to see who's the fastest runner, who has the most."

Compared to the years before the Cuban crisis, when it was possible to acquire most foods, clothes, and household goods at a low price, there is now almost nothing to share for those without access to U.S. dollars. Cuba is becoming a class society (Zimbalist 2000:13) and is divided into those who earn local-currency pesos and those who have access to dollars. Those with dollars can enjoy shopping centers and supermarkets with both locally made and imported goods, while for most people living on a salary in pesos, life is a struggle from day to day. This situation has created envy and hard feelings, and many, both religious devotees and others, know someone who has been the victim of some evil work.

A "Life Switch" Case

As sorcery is said to have become more common through the years of the economic crisis, hospital treatments that do not turn out well are also sometimes explained as an act of sorcery. It is common to perform some kind of protective santería ritual at home or inside the hospital so as to avoid picking up some bad thing from someone else. One example of the kind of sorcery in which something bad or evil is sent from one person to another is known as a *cambio de vida* (life switch).

The life switch can take place between a person and a doll or animal, but in hospitals it often takes place between two patients. The illness or weak "life" of a sick, dying patient is taken away and put into an almost healthy person. The illness of the sick person is exchanged for the health or life of the healthy one. As a result the person ready to leave the hospital becomes very ill or dies, and the formerly dying person is healed and walks out of the hospital. This magic is performed easily between two people with beds close to each other in the same room.

In one life switch case, a woman in her forties came to a hospital because she was suffering from a heavy cold. In the bed in front of her, another very ill, dying woman was visited by people who carried out different kinds of magical work. After two weeks the formerly dying woman was up on her feet and could leave the hospital. The woman supposedly suffering from the cold became worse, and the doctors discovered that she had lung cancer. A santería priest found out through divination that she had been the victim of a life switch. She was told that she would become well if she carried out certain santería rituals, which she did. She also had to do a spiritual mass for her dead ancestors and a mass in the church. The woman's condition apparently improved slightly.

Even if, in this case, further divination indicates that the cancer will continue, the santero may recommend initiation to alleviate the suffering. She may also be told that her time on earth has come to an end and that there is very little that can be done. A life switch is generally considered a powerful kind of work, and it is difficult to do much against it. An extract from a conversation about life switching with A.M., a physician and babalao, shows some of the difficulties but also possibilities, when biomedicine and magic meet:

J.W.: As a religious practitioner you can believe in the life switch, but as a physician you are not supposed to believe that this really exists?

A.M.: It exists, it can be done. As a physician I cannot say that, but for myself I can think like that. I would never do it with another person, that is a bad thing, and it is only carried out by people without scruples. I would do it with an animal that would take over the illness from the person.

J.W.: What is your reaction if you suspect that someone has carried out a life switch in the hospital?

A.M.: If I see that an almost healthy person becomes very ill and dies, and the one in the next bed who suffered from a serious illness rapidly becomes well, and that the relatives carried out some rituals, I will be very surprised as a physician. As a babalao I will not be surprised. I would say, "They worked well."

J.W.: Do you find it difficult to work as both a babalao and a physician?

A.M.: When I work as a physician it is difficult to think as a babalao, although it happens that I use my religion and ask [through divination] about the illness of a patient. Every day I ask Orula to help me diagnose when I work as a physician. When I work as a babalao it's easier, as I can speak more openly as both a physician and a babalao. In the last case, if the person has problems with a social origin, I can take care of it as a babalao, and if it is a physical illness I can both treat him with my religious knowledge and recommend [Western] medical treatment.

Sorcery clearly has an existential dimension. When illness is expressed in terms of sorcery, it can be seen both as a commentary on the victim's social situation and as part of the human condition. Through the discourse of sorcery, a reason for illness and suffering is given (cf. Thylefors 2002). Sorcery is both "a metaphor for the chaos that constitutes social relations" (Stoller and Olkes 1987:229) and a vehicle of change, opening up the possibility for human beings to change the circumstances of their lives (cf. Kapferer 1997:21).

In order to protect and heal himself and others from illness caused by sorcery or by something else, the santero needs to have practical knowledge of the santería rituals and of all kinds of minor trabajos. He must also learn how to interpret his dreams. A santero explained: "Through dreams I receive messages of how to heal a person. A spirit may come and tell me which plants to use or may say, 'Take this chicken and cleanse this person in order to take away the badness.' The santos may also reveal themselves in dreams and tell you what to do, and you may even open your eyes and see them. They come as Catholic images or you may dream about a person possessed with a santo who will tell you what to do."

The santero needs to know how to communicate with, and relate to, the santería divinities through offerings, sacrifices, ritual cleansings, possession trance, prayers, music, dance, and dreams. All these activities are part of the healing process, which, in turn, is based on communication with the divinities; humans perform divine works and are given health, luck, and prosperity in return.

Responses to Illness

In order to create balance and harmony, avoid illness, or restore health, sacrifices are carried out. The concept of ebbó is crucial in all kinds of rituals. It is performed as a means of communicating with the divine world, neutralizing sorcery and evil, and gaining strength, help, and protection. Ebbó can consist of lighting a candle or offering food to the santos. It can also mean animal sacrifice and the sprinkling of blood over ritual objects, in particular, the sacred stones that represent the santos.

The stones, which contain large amounts of divine power, are normally kept in large soup tureens of porcelain or ceramic. When not in use they are put on a shelf in the canastillero (a shelved cabinet) with other objects that represent the santo. According to Brandon (1990:126f), ebbó is santería's "answer to the problem of suffering, a means to achieve harmony in a universe composed of teeming forces . . . [and] [t]hrough the medium of ebo [ebbó] . . . the disordered universe is replaced by freshness, clarity, and peace."

The santos need to be "fed" with blood to exist. They have to "eat." In turn they give ashé to humans. When sacrifices are carried out, ashé is released. To restore balance through sacrifice can therefore be said to be the fundamental form of illness treatment in santería. It would be of no use to expect to become healed from a severe illness before spiritual balance has been restored.

Blood from sacrificed animals is considered very powerful. Ashé is released when blood is poured over the sacred stones and other objects that represent the santos. It is not the blood as such, however, that contains power. The blood must come from an animal that is being sacrificed. A santería priest from Matanzas told me with aversion that "in the U.S. the santeros now even buy bottles with blood instead of killing animals. That is not the way it should be done." The exchange by which humans give blood to the santos, who reciprocate by giving strength and health in the form of ashé, was expressed by another santero who said: "Blood gives vitality, it gives life. Therefore we have to sacrifice animals." Death gives life.

The role of blood in sacrifice also becomes apparent when someone is going through surgery in a hospital. In this case the animal that is to be sacrificed may be kept alive until after the medical operation. The santería divinity that is said to be responsible for the operation is promised the blood from the animal after the operation. This is done to ensure that the divinity will give its help during the whole process but also because "blood calls blood," meaning that a release of blood during sacrifice can cause a similar loss of blood during surgery at a hospital. For the same reason, menstruating women are not supposed to participate in rituals where animals are sacrificed.

When a person suffers from an ailment because of lack of ashé, there exists an imbalance that must be redressed by using "hot" and "cool" liquids and objects. The hot-cool distinction is an old and widespread concept that also can be found in many healing theories in Europe, Asia, and Latin America (Voeks 1997:130f). In santería, blood is generally considered hot, and when blood is poured over ritual objects, everything has to be covered with feathers from fowl, as feathers are cool and fresh. Water is also considered fresh and is sprinkled over the objects. When a divination session is about to begin, coolness is emphasized as the priest says in Lucumí: "Fresh water, fresh road ["way of life"], fresh money, freshness for the children, long life, life through almighty father" (Valdés Garriz 1997:126). The divinities can also be classified as either hot or cool, with the exception of the trickster divinity Eleggua. Accordingly, Shangó, Ogún, Aggayú, and Oyá are said to be hot, while Oshún, Obatalá, Yemayá, Osain, and Ochosi are considered cool.

The power of the santero emanates from his ashé (divine power), and it is said that a santero with many godchildren has a lot of ashé. The term ashé also means "luck," "health," and "prosperity," which will follow when a close relationship to the divine world of the santos is developed and maintained. The devotee will live a healthier life and be warned of impending illnesses and will have more luck finding a job, fewer problems with the police, greater success when competing with others, and so on.

On one occasion, a santero presented me to one of his godchildren who "was nothing before." Today, thanks to initiation and the powers of the santos, he is the manager of a large school. My friend Julio, a babalao from Havana, has many clients and godchildren. He explained: "If I have ashé I don't have to go to other people's houses and live from them. Instead, people come here and the house is always full of people. Thus, I resolve people's problems, and they give me things so I can resolve my own problems. This is called ashé, luck."

The economic situation of the babalao or santero improves even more markedly if the clients are foreigners. Some santeros and babalao priests, especially in Havana, make a considerable profit by divining and carrying out rituals for tourists and other foreign visitors. Some of the most successful priests frequently travel to neighboring countries to carry out initiations. They may have a large network of godchildren who send cash, medicines, and gifts. This is considered evidence of the priest's large quantity of ashé, which, in turn, may lead to more godchildren.

All Cubans have suffered deeply from the years of the economic crisis and have experienced great changes in their society. Social networks have become increasingly important because life has become more competitive. People often claimed that one needs to have a godfather to solve one's problems. They told me how important it had become to have informal contacts and relations with all kinds of people. A desperately needed medicine that is out of stock is obtained by a friend who works in the pharmacy. An appointment for surgery becomes possible despite long queues if one knows the doctor. An attractive job in the tourist industry is achieved through the right contacts, and so on.

The crisis is altering the norms of sharing and mutual aid that prevailed in Cuban society before the crisis. Now, people cannot afford to help each other as they did before. Many feel powerless to control their own lives. By becoming initiated into santería, however, the situation changes. Through the initiation ritual, a bond to the world of the santería divinities is created. The initiate now comes under the protection of a certain santo that has been made, as well as by some other santos that have been received.

The devotee is also ritually linked to a *padrino* or *madrina* through the initiation ritual and can request help from them. To turn down such a request would offend not only humans but also the santos. Similarly, a godchild is obliged to help his godfather or godmother. On one occasion, for example, when the son of a powerful santero was arrested, the santero picked up the phone and called two of his godchildren who are police chiefs. They assured him that they personally would take care of the problem. (This particular time the police chiefs did not have to interfere; the santero's son was released anyway. His crime had been to cycle against the traffic without an owner's certificate for the bicycle.)

The fact that social and political power easily transforms into divine power, and vice versa, is explicit in the discourse on the Cuban leader, Fidel Castro. Both santeros and babalaos assured me that his power, and the fact that he maintained it, was due to the religious ceremonies and the initiations that he had made. On a visit to Africa, they said, he went through really powerful work. Only this could explain his outstanding strength. As one santero said, "If he wasn't protected, how could he survive all the attempts that have been made to kill him?"

Beauty and the Power of Music and Dance

In santería, the success of major rituals is related to the aesthetic aspects of the objects, clothes, and the performance involved. A successful ritual is often said to be *linda* or *bonita*, beautiful. On these occasions an altar is made for the santo the devotee has made, and for the other santos that have been received. Offerings of fruits, cakes, and flowers are placed on the altar together with the *soperas* (soup tureens) that contain the sacred stones. Each sopera is covered with a fine shiny cloth *(pañuelo)*, in colors appropriate to each of the santos being celebrated.

The plastic bead necklaces, each with combinations of colors that correspond to particular santos, are laid over the soperas. Other objects related to each of the devotee's santos, like Shangó's wooden double ax or Oshún's fan, are also put on the altar. The ceremony and the altar are first and foremost for the santos, which becomes evident when people arrive. First they go directly to the altar and salute the santos. Standing on their knees they ring a little bell and put some money in a bowl in front of the altar. Then they greet the other participants in the ceremony.

When building and displaying an altar, the aesthetic aspects are important for creating and maintaining a relationship with the santos. The process of building an altar is time consuming and often expensive. Many save for months, and those who have relatives abroad ask them to bring or send a nice shiny cloth for the celebration. A new cloth should preferably be used each year, something that few can afford. A large altar with new cloths and other objects suggests that the santero is prosperous and has many godchildren. More importantly, though, to build an aesthetically appropriate altar is a way to participate in a series of exchanges with the santos. The devotee is protected and helped by the santos, who, in turn, are offered a beautiful altar (Brown 1996; cf. Lawal 1996:11).

Santeros often pointed out to me that giving to the santos should never be performed with self-interest. A devotee shows her or his relationship and gratitude to the santos through love. To give "from the heart," by making the altar as beautiful as possible, is the best way to show this devotion. It is the willingness to give that matters most, not the money put into the building of the altar.

When I attended "birthday" ceremonies or other feasts, I often heard people say, "Shangó will like this," or "Oshún will be very pleased," even though the altars were small and simple. The participants said that such altars were beautifully arranged, despite the poverty of the santero who was performing the celebration. It is important that an altar be aesthetically pleasing and reflect the characteristics of the santo being honored. An altar for Shangó, for example, should correspond to his masculinity, while an altar for Oshún "must convey the distinctive values associated with a goddess of love, sweetness, and sensuality" (Flores-Peña and Evanchuk 1994:15).

Equally important are the music and dance performed during rituals. The initiate experiences new ways of moving and feeling the body when singing and dancing to the sacred drums and when paying respect to other santeros and santería altars by prostrating himself or herself on the floor (Mason 1994). Worshippers often relate their experience to recitations, music, song, and dance of a major ritual. When the divine power in speech, music, and dance come together in the ritual, ashé will be released and will strengthen the participants.

Speech and song are also important in rituals. Before all forms of divination, the santos are invoked by prayers in Lucumí, a practice called *moyub-bar*. Similarly, when sacrifices are carried out, the priest sings in the ritual language. To speak, pray, and sing in Lucumí during rituals means to liberate ashé. Words expressed in Lucumí have ashé. These words empower the participants and therefore not only "say something" but also "do something."

Priests and other participants also sing in Lucumí, often about events from santería mythology, while dancing to the beat of the drums during a ceremony. The *oriaté* (song leader) and the participants sing and follow the beat of the drums in a complex interplay that goes on for hours. The cer-

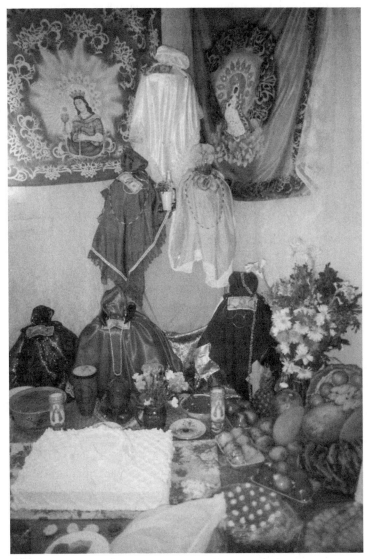

Fig. 10. Flowers, cakes, and fruits offered to the santos during a "birthday" ceremony. Shiny cloths cover the soup tureens where the sacred stones are kept. Photo by Johan Wedel.

emony usually takes place in a specially prepared room in a private house. Since it is open to all who want to come, it is usually very crowded.

The three sacred *batá* drums used for an initiation contain a large amount of ashé that is released when they are played. The largest, the "mother," is called Iyá, the middle Itótele, and the smallest Okónkolo. The musicians are seated with the drums, two-headed and hourglass shaped, placed horizontally on their knees. The construction of the drums is a complicated and highly secret process that involves omiero, animal sacrifices, and divination to the spirit Aña, who resides in the largest drum. The "voice" from baptized drums must also be passed over to the new ones. When consecrated, they are considered to be very powerful, with their own will (see also Castellanos and Castellanos 1994:308).

According to Benkomo (2000:142), "The drum is an *orisha*. It has its birthday, it eats, it has to be initiated with coconut. It has a life of its own. . . . There are times when it's tired, when it doesn't want to work." During an initiation, the drums play a central role, and the initiate dances to the beat of the drums on the "day of the presentation." According to a santero, "The initiate dances in front of the drums so that the drums' spirit will recognize that the person has made santo."

The drumbeat, which is very complex and takes many years to learn, follows a predetermined ritual order called Oru that always opens and closes with an evocation to Eleggua, the santo that opens and closes roads and pathways. Other santos are then called upon with their distinct rhythms and songs. The rhythms evoke the character and temper appropriate to each of the santos. More importantly, these sacred rhythms not only evoke and represent the santos; the ashé of the divinities is also present in the sound of the drums.

Music is heard in the body, and dance is the extension of music. The presence of the santos is felt in the body of the participants through the medium of the music. During a drum ceremony *(tambor)*, the santeros dance in front of the three drum players. By dancing, the santeros approach a "cosmic unity" with the divinity that they conjure up through their movements. Dressed like kings or queens in the clothes and colors of the santo they have made, they dance according to the mythological characteristics of their santo.

Possession Trance

As the santeros dance, and if the drums are played in the right manner accompanied by song to create an intense atmosphere, the santos will be attracted and will possess their human "children." It is said that the santo "mounts" *(monta)* the santero; it "comes down" or "descends" *(baja),* or "ascends" *(sube).* The first time a person becomes possessed, usually during initiation, the possessed is partially conscious of what happens. When complete trance takes place, the santero, possessed with the santo and completely unaware of what is happening, will continue to dance but in a much more intense and powerful way.

I was often amazed by how people changed, not only mentally but also physically, when the santo descended; the face of a young man could suddenly look fifteen or twenty years older, an old woman could become strong and agile. The divinities, in possession of their human hosts, perform extraordinary dances and actions and advise humans about their health and life situation. During the ceremonies in which I participated, santería priests who were possessed by santos often recommended that participants see a doctor or carry out some kind of sacrifice or cleansing of evil influences when confronted with a health problem.

When dancing, each santo has its own movements and style; Eleggua dances with a red and black *garabato* (hooked staff); Shangó raises his hand, symbolically touching flashes of lightning in the sky while swinging his red double ax and sticking out his tongue as a symbol of fire; Oshún dances with a fan, as does Yemayá, who moves like the waves in the sea; Obba dances with her hand covering one of her ears, enacting the myth where she was fooled into cutting off her ear; Ogún swings a machete; and Ochosi's movements recall a hunter shooting arrows. The initiates gradually learn these movements as they participate in rituals. When the santeros dance, possessed by the santos, ashé is liberated in the movements of the dance, in the Lucumí songs, and through the beat of the drums.

The santos who possess their devotees not only dance but can also cleanse everybody from bad influences, with smoke, water, herbs, or other objects. If someone is suffering from an illness in a certain part of the body, the person possessed by the santo passes a hand over the afflicted area. The santería divinities will also give individual advice about illness and social relations. The participants present are therefore in different ways affected by the ashé that the santos carry with them. Possession, then, conveys the power that gives life and health.

When the santo comes down, the devotee usually begins to shake and tremble furiously. Gradually, as the divinity mounts, the devotee becomes calm. Possession trance, it appears, is no playacting. The dancer is removed from the reality of everyday life and will not remember anything of what happened during possession. Although music and dance are important for invoking possession trance, it may also take place on other occasions. This is rare, but suggests that these media are not a prerequisite for possession, even if they are closely related. Generally, music itself does not induce trance, but as the santos descend and possess humans and, thus, give of their ashé, the drumbeat suggests that hearing is also an important sense in rituals.

The experience of possession trance was explained by a santería priest as "falling into something empty" or as "a sensation that makes you leave this world." Participants often told me how they became dizzy during the intense drumming and singing and experienced a sensation of leaving their bodies. Many also expressed joy and relief from previous problems when the ritual was over.

Discussing the intense atmosphere during santería ceremonies in the United States, Canizares (1993:73) tells how participants often experience "an inexplicable outpouring of energy similar to the power of an erupting volcano." Murphy (1993:98) relates how he is "lifted, called, carried by the rhythm, alternating between anxiety at the strange sensations and deep calm because the flow is strong and sure." He feels relaxed and "things seem very slow indeed and crystal clear."

Anthropologists working in other parts of the world have had similar experiences. In Zambia, Willis (1999:116) relates how, during two Lungu ceremonies involving drumming, he "had the very distinct sense of being in a changed state of consciousness, in which the ordinary-reality parameters of 'time' and 'space' had somehow been dissolved." He felt "'lifted' out of normal reality into a condition of pleasurably heightened awareness, which could fairly be called one of mild ecstasy." Similarly, during a ritual among the Tumbaka in Malawi, Friedson (1996:18) danced to the singing, clapping, and drumming when his "body just sort of took over and followed the distinct rhythmic motto of the *umphanda* spirits." His "perception was becoming detached" from his body as if he was "watching someone else dance."

While clapping to the drumming during a Ndembu healing ritual in Zambia, E. Turner (1992:149) had a profound spiritual experience: "A certain palpable social integument broke and something *calved* along with me. I felt the spiritual motion, a tangible feeling of breakthrough going through the whole group. . . . [The body became] deeply involved in the rhythm." According to E. Turner (74), "Trance follows a sudden consciousness of pure knowledge, the 'I know' syndrome. . . . The outside world fades, pain does not pain, time is not time, human will is left behind."

Ritually induced trance is a feature common to many societies all over the world and possibly a near-universal capacity (Bourguignon 1973). Experiments suggest that repetitive auditory stimuli, such as ritual drumming, may affect the human central nervous system, especially the right hemisphere of the brain. The mode of thought in the right cerebral hemisphere is said to be related to emotions and holistic thinking, but linguistic capacity is limited and the perception of time is absent. This may explain why participants often feel strong emotions and experience unusual, timeless, inexpressible sensations during rituals involving drumming (Neher 1962; Lex 1979; V. Turner 1985). When testing physiological reactions during trance, Goodman (1988:39, 1990:25) found an increase in the heart rate and a simultaneous drop in blood pressure, a finding associated with near-death. The reaction was accompanied by a drop in the compounds that indicate stress (such as adrenaline) in the blood serum, the appearance of endorphins (the body's painkiller), and electrical brain activity otherwise seen only before sleep or during deep Zen meditation.

The physiological aspects of possession may bring some clarity to the phenomenon, but the individual experience of possession trance must also be understood and related to the quality of the ritual taking place: the skill of the drummers; the specific "atmosphere" and intensity of the performance; and relations between the drummers and between them and the other participants (see Willis 1999:117ff).

During one santería ritual in Matanzas that I attended, a man in his early forties was initiated and had made Shangó. He had suffered from pain in his stomach and thought he had a stomach ulcer, but he said the doctors were not sure. During the itá (divination) it was confirmed that he really had a stomach ulcer. He was advised to go back for a medical examination and was told that this time, thanks to the initiation, the doctors would now "see clear" and give him the correct treatment. On the first day of his initiation, he already began to feel better, he explained. He drank much omiero, and over the following days he felt a great calmness.

On the fourth day, the day of presentation, he was presented for the sacred batá drums. The ceremony took place in the backyard of his godmother's house. About fifty people had gathered, and the three drum players were sitting with the decorated drums on their knees. The initiate, who was addressed as iyabó by everyone, sat on his throne in the cuarto de santo, a small house close to the yard. Beside him stood the objects of Shangó: a round wooden container and a double ax. The iyabó wore a beautifully ornamented dress and had a painted face and a crown on his head. As the drummers played, accompanied by song, those present who were santeros began to dance in a circle.

After about a half hour the drumming became more intense, and the santeros lined up in two rows in front of the cuarto de santo. They held raised sticks with a red ribbon in their hands and formed a "roof."[2] As the music intensified, the iyabó finally came out. Escorted by an elder santero, he walked slowly under the sticks toward the drummers on the other side of the yard. He kissed the drums, lay down in front of the largest one, and then rose and begun to dance. He looked dizzy but was not possessed. After about fifteen minutes he was led back to the small room while the other santeros continued to dance.

Suddenly, a girl in her early twenties who had recently become initiated, wearing white clothes and a white headdress, became possessed with her santo, Obatalá. She transformed completely. Her young face was now that of a very old woman. She had great difficulty standing upright, and she was breathing heavily. An old "aspect" of Obatalá had taken over her body, and she danced slowly. As the drumming continued, the song leader urged the participants to sing louder. "Are you dumb?" he asked. The atmosphere was now intense, and people became possessed. Oshún "took over" a middle-aged woman. With wide-open eyes, she laughed and gave advice to all present in a combination of Spanish and Lucumí, and an interpreter translated her words.

When it was my turn to meet her, she told me that I knew more about santería than I would admit and that I therefore should "make santo." She smeared honey on my hands, and I in turn smeared it on my neck and in my face. I was also told to put my sticky hands in my pockets. "This means money. Money will come to you," a santero and friend of mine said, and added with a laugh, "Make sure that I receive some of it, too!"

The Use of Plants and Herbs in Healing

Knowledge about herbs and plants and how to use them in healing has been important in Cuba for a long time. Dianteill (2000:287, 297), for example, mentions a santería manual said to be a copy of an original dated January 16, 1836. It contains a list of the most important herbs and plants used in the religion, and these are classified according to the divinities who are said to "own" them. In a pragmatic way, the manual also describes different kinds of offerings and works.

The herbal knowledge described in the manual is no less important today. Afro-Cuban herbalists know the healing properties "of hundreds of trees, roots, barks, grasses, herbs, vines and flowers" (Marks 1987:229). The role of herbs and plants is often emphasized by the santería priests. Herbs and plants are said to be indispensable in all kinds of rituals, and the santero needs to know both the natural and supernatural properties of herbs and plants. This knowledge forms part of the santero's healing knowledge:

"Those plants that do not help through some pharmacological efficacy are thought to help through the efficacy of their magical powers" (Brandon 1991:58). Many santería priests have a vast knowledge of herbs and plants, and, depending on the form of illness and its origin, they prescribe different treatments. In the case of stomach problems, inflammations, skin problems, or headaches and fevers, treatment may be carried out with herbs outside of the religious context.

Highly valued is the sacred ceiba tree (see app. 1). In one myth the ceiba saved the world from annihilation; in another it taught Orula the secrets of divination. The ceiba is said to have great divine powers, and sacrifices are often put at the foot of the tree. For a spiritual bath against illness in general, leaves from the ceiba tree and the salvadera plant are ripped and mixed with honey, cascarilla, perfume, and dry wine.

The coconut, which is owned by Obatalá, is also of great importance. It is used in all rituals and in divination. The santería priest Benedí, who was interviewed by Lewis and his team (Lewis et al. 1977a:61), explained how he came to a house where a man was very ill. He divined with the coconuts and asked if he could use the herb romerillo to heal the person. The answer was yes, and it was mixed together with dry wine and honey and given to the patient. According to Benedí, the patient recovered. In a famous myth, it is told how *obí*, the coconut, became a divination tool when the supreme god Olofi punished obí for his arrogant and dominant attitude:

In the old days the coconut was all white, both inside and outside. He was a wealthy and proud man because he was white and lived like a king. But he was also vain and contemptuous of all people, and he treated them very badly and was despotic. One day a beggar came, raised his hand, and asked for money. Obí pushed him away with indignation and disgust, saying to him that he did not want to touch him because he was very dirty. The supreme god Olofi saw what was happening and said to obí: "Because of your scornfulness and your vanity, from this moment you will live miserably on the floor, and one part of you will be black and the other white. From now on you must humbly serve all humans and all divinities." That's why the coconut is thrown on the floor when it's used for divination.

There are several versions of this myth, but in all of them obí is punished for his arrogance. According to Cabrera (1993a:381), the coconut is an agent for interrupting an illness, but it can also be used to destroy a person. The coconut is smashed at a crossroads as the person says, "The same way as I break this coconut, the illness of X will be broken," or "Just as I break this coconut, the life, house, and fate of so-and-so will be broken." Interestingly, the word "crossroads," used by Cabrera, is the Spanish *encrucijada,* which, according to the dictionary *Cuyás* (1960), also means "chance to do harm to another" or "ambush."

Plants, weeds, and herbs are indispensable in all kinds of rituals because they contain ashé. In the ritual context, they are seen as sacred and as living things with different characteristics. "Some are easily frightened and there-fore withhold their powers by refusing to bloom. Others are retiring and shy. Others have brittle, explosive personalities and require the utmost in eti-quette and respect before being picked. If not pampered, others will simply hide the next time you want to find them" (Brandon 1991:58).

When plants and herbs are bought at the yerbero for use in santería ritu-als, the santero must know that they were picked in the right way, or else they will be powerless. They must be collected by *osainistas* (experts on herbs and plants). When the osainistas enter the forest where Osain, the lord of plants and herbs, reigns, they offer maize, liquor, and smoke from a cigar. Before picking the plants, they must first ask them for permission, pay them a tribute, and sing to them. These osainistas do not have to be santeros or santeras, but they must have a profound knowledge of herbs and plants and their characteristics.

Osain is also the name of an herbal concoction used during initiation into santería. The mixture, which is made while the participants sing to the plants, contains a minimum of twenty-one different plants that may vary according to the divinities involved in the ritual. Distinct osains are made for each divinity. While singing and crushing the herbs, the santeros trans-fer some of their ashé to the mixture, which is then used for washing the religious objects (Brandon 1991:60).

Parts of the respective osains are set apart and later poured into a com-mon bowl. This mixture, which also contains water from a coconut, or rain-water from the month of May, is called omiero. It is given to the initiate to bathe in and to drink, and all the religious objects of the initiate are also washed in the mixture. It is considered very fresh, revitalizing, powerful, and strengthening because it contains large amounts of ashé and is also said to kill bacteria and prevent illness. Further, during santería initiation, differ-ent plants and herbs are used to make a powder, also called ashé, which is said to protect the initiate from illness.

Without Osain, the lord of all the plants and herbs in the forest, there are no rites, no magic, and no medicine, according to Cabrera (1993a:106). He is the source, the healer who gives ashé from god Olofi to all the santos, and he knows all the secrets of the forest. He is also the guardian of the sacred batá drums, which are used during the initiation ritual. The relationship between Osain and the batá drums is explained in a myth in which the chief of the animals in the forest was very ill and was therefore playing the batá drums. Osain cured him with his herbs and was taught the secret of playing the drums in return (Pérez Medina 1998:377).

Osain administers and distributes the plants and gives the plants needed to heal or to bring sickness upon someone (Cabrera 1993a:101), though each of the other santos are also related to, and considered owners of, certain plants. The plants rompezaragüey and salvadera, for example, are owned by Shangó. Canutillo is owned by Yemayá, while berro belongs to Oshún.

All the herbs and plants belong to a certain santo. This "folk taxonomy involving orisha ownership" (Marks 1987:228) is grounded in a logic that also includes parts of the human body. A healing practice involving the santo Oshún illustrates the relation between a santería divinity, a certain plant, and a distinctive part of the human body. Oshún is related to the womb and is the owner of the calabash. Accordingly, when someone has a problem with the womb, a pumpkin is passed over the afflicted area together with honey, which is also related to Oshún. The sunflower is also owned by Oshún and may be used in a similar way. It is also used for holding spirits at bay, and a mixture made from its leaves is utilized for vaginal douches.

Another example is the plant escoba amarga. The plant belongs to San Lazaro, the great healer of illness and the ruler of smallpox, leprosy, and all kinds of skin diseases. The plant is often used against pustules on the skin. When someone is about to die of an illness, escoba amarga is also used in a spiritual bath. It is mixed together with salvia, which is also owned by San Lazaro, and with salvadera. The decoction is poured over the body seven times over seven days in order to chase away death (Ikú). In another bath against serious illness that may result in death, almácigo, granada, cascarilla, and dried meat from fish and from a kind of ferret are boiled together and poured over the body seven times over seven days while praying to Oyá, who is related to death, and Obatalá, who is related to calmness and stability.

Obatalá is the owner of the white cotton bush. The divinity is associated with calmness, stability, peace, whiteness, purity, and cleanliness. A decoction of the seeds of the cotton bush is used against bronchitis, asthma, and head lice. The luster of its flowers will eliminate evil eye and work against immorality and other "impure" human acts. Its leaves are also important ingredients when making the omiero for the initiation ritual.

Based on studies by Cabrera (1993a) and Ayensu (1981), Marks (1987) also discusses the use of the cotton bush and other herbs and plants in santería. He argues that santería's classification of herbs and plants may constitute pharmacological categories and that santería herbalists "may have discovered what the ethnobotanists' chemical analyses are now revealing" (Marks 1987:231). From the cotton bush, an oil can be extracted that contains salicylic acid, which has bacteriostatic action. The plant is recommended by santería priests for use in baths for persons with poor hygiene, which may cause health problems. A further example is the tree jía brava that belongs to the Flacourtia family. San Lazaro owns this tree. Two other trees that belong to the same family are used in the treatment of leprosy elsewhere in the Caribbean, and, according to Marks (235), it is probable that jia brava has similar properties.

Because practicing santería priests have a great deal of knowledge of medicinal plants and are known to heal illness related to the spirit-world, they are often consulted after the patient has made a visit to a physician. The plants álamo, sasafrás, and yerba mora, for example, may be used to treat problems caused by sorcery. Many plants and herbs are used today by both santería priests and physicians in Cuba. The use of mastuerzo is one example. The plant is often used by both categories in cases of kidney problems. In santería, mastuerzo is also used in the "rogation of the head" ritual, to strengthen the client's memory. Another example is sábila, which is recommended by many physicians and santeros in cases of vaginal inflammations.

The use of herbs and plants in santería is based on empirically observed results, and many of the plant medicines probably contain pharmacologically active chemicals. Their physiological efficacy, however, also depends on how they are prepared, combined, and administered (see also Etkin 1996). As with all therapies involving herbs and plants, they "are effective if they effect or assist in producing the requisite, culturally defined outcomes" (Etkin 1988:301).

Knowing how to use plant medicines is an important part of santería healing knowledge, but the plants and herbs do not always have to be in contact with the human body to heal, cleanse, protect, and expel bad magic. As a general prophylaxis against illness, items such as an ear of corn wrapped in a bundle of purple ribbons may be placed behind the door. According to Brandon (1991:64f), the inhabitants of a house may protect themselves against sorcery by spreading petals of galán de día in the house or placing okra over the door of the house. All the outside doors may also be washed with guásima, and bushes of ruda may be planted near each door.

These ways of administering plants and herbs are thought to expel evil influences and promote health and well-being, even though the plants never actually come into contact with the human body and cannot therefore have any direct physiological effect. Galán de día, for example, which is owned by Obatalá, is said to purify the house and create a happy environment (Cabrera 1993a:408).

It is important to have knowledge of these protective plants since there are many ways to bring illness and misfortune to the people of a household. In one such "work," Dianteill (2000:300) relates how a mixture of sulfur, mustard seeds, peppercorn, and the plant rascabarriga is placed in three eggs. These are placed next to Eleggua for three days before a Friday or Monday. Two of the eggs are then thrown at the two street corners closest to the house, while the third is thrown in front of the door of the victim's house.

When sorcery is directed toward a specific household, all the people living in the house may be affected. I was myself involved in one such case in Matanzas when the family in the house next to where I lived was exposed to sorcery. The family had received some money from a relative abroad and was renovating their house. During the final weeks, however, things began to go wrong. The mother of the house fell down the stairs and hurt her knee. Her nerves were also bad. Some of the construction material was stolen, and the workers did not show up. Further, the mother claimed she sometimes heard a noise on the roof, although nobody was up there.

One morning, the family woke up and found that someone had thrown pepper in front of the main door. The family's fears seemed justified, as pepper is often used in evil works. It was no coincidence that everything had gone wrong; someone was performing sorcery against them. A friend who is also a santero explained that it was probably a neighbor who had sent a dark spirit on the house and thrown the pepper at the door. The reason was said to be envy.

I went to an open field with the santero to find the right herbs to counter the spirit attack. We picked a few bundles of rompezaragüey and cleansed all the walls in the house with the herbs, which were then hung from the ceiling. After the cleansing, everybody in the house was relieved. The mother's nerves improved, and after a few days the construction work recommenced.

The following case, which involves biomedicine, spiritism, and santería, gives an example of how herbs can be applied to the body. A young girl was suffering from the disease optic neuritis because of vitamin deficiency. She had incorrectly used an herbal cream prescribed by a physician, and by the time she visited a person who worked as both a spiritist and santería priestess, her eyesight had been impaired. During the consultation the spiritist/santería priestess became possessed by her muerto.

The muerto told the girl's parents to interrupt the treatment ordered by the physician and prescribed instead other herbs. She also performed a limpieza. The spirit said that the girl had to go through medio asiento, a santería halfway initiation that is a ceremony often aimed at restoring health. The ceremony is done as fast as possible when there is no time to prepare for the complete seven-day initiation. The medio asiento includes sacrifices and a washing of the sick person's head and body with a mixture of crushed herbs. Shortly after the rituals the disorder ceased.

Divine power or force of life, ashé, is vital when explaining, avoiding, and responding to an affliction. Illness is often related to a lack of ashé and spiritual imbalance. When animals are sacrificed, ashé is released as the divinities "eat" and health is restored. A priest who has much ashé is financially successful and spiritually powerful and has many godchildren. His success is considered evidence of his ashé, which also protects him against sorcery attacks from people who want to hurt him by sending an illness or other misfortune on him. In this view, illness is often considered to have been caused by supernatural agents; it is related to the social world of the sufferer through a discourse of sorcery.

If rituals are to be successful and the divinities are to give of their ashé to humans, altars must be made in a beautiful way. If ashé is to be released and the divinities descend, the sacred drums, which also contain ashé, must be played in the right way, together with prayers and song. Through possession trance, the divinities possess humans and give of their ashé in order to bring health and prosperity to the participants. Ashé is also present in sacred stones and in herbs and plants if they are picked in the right manner. Through the presence of ashé in offerings, sacrifices, music, possession trance, objects, and herbs and plants, the sufferer is empowered, healing is achieved, and illness is prevented.

4

Pantheon and Rituals

The Santería Pantheon

In Africa, hundreds of deities (orishas) can be found in the Yoruba pantheon. Many of these were worshipped in a particular region in Yorubaland. Others, like Ogún, lord of iron, and Obatalá, lord of peace and purity, were well known and worshipped all over the territory. Only a few of the more widely known orishas survived in Cuba. In this new setting, beliefs in the orishas were transformed and elements from Roman Catholicism were borrowed. The orishas are archetypes, divine forces of nature with human characteristics. They are usually called santos (saints), and almost all of them have a Catholic correspondence that may, or may not, be of the opposite sex. The characters of the santos are discussed here in their most general and commonly used forms. For the devotee, the different aspects of the santos must also be taken into consideration.

Belief in the orishas/santos is accompanied by hundreds of myths *(patakies)* and proverbs. Initiates learn about the religion by listening when experienced santeros narrate myths. Many of these myths deal with problems faced by orishas/santos, heroes, and other spiritual beings, and how the problems were resolved. Other myths discuss the origin of certain rites and prohibitions, or the creation of the world, of humans, and of animals. A moral intention is frequently present, and the santos commonly act like humans, with their weaknesses. Often the myths emphasize a need to carry out a sacrifice, and they explain what happens when the prescribed sacrifice is, or is not, carried out.

Santería does not constitute an entirely coherent body of beliefs and rituals, and practices may vary considerably. However, all devotees share a general understanding of the characteristics of the most common divinities. Most important is Olodumare, the supreme god and creator of the universe. He is also known as Olorun and is often personified in myths as Olofi. He is a very remote god and takes little interest in human affairs. According to one myth, the god distributed his ashé to the orishas/santos. Thus, the santos have their origin in the ashé that comes from Olodumare. The ashé, in turn, is crucial in all human activities. As humans develop a relationship with the santos and become their "children," they benefit from the ashé emitted by Olodumare.

Obatalá, king and father of the other santos, completed the creation on earth. In a well-known myth, he modeled man from clay. Obatalá is the ruler of the head and the lord of purity, peace, justice, and patience. He is revered for his great healing powers (Sandoval 1995:86). It is said that he is the owner of the head, and he rules over the eyesight. The color related to Obatalá is white, and the objects that represent him are kept in a high place, covered in cotton. He is usually identified with the Catholic saint Our Lady of Mercy. Children of Obatalá are said to be tranquil, patient, and peaceful. The relationship between peacefulness and the divinity Obatalá became apparent when Pope John Paul II visited Cuba in January 1998. Several santería priests told me that he was a child of Obatalá, because of his peacefulness and patience. In this myth about human nature, narrated by a santero from Matanzas, Obatalá serves a dish to Olofi.

> Once upon a time Olofi, the supreme god, old, tired, and far from the human world, asked Obatalá, the orisha of peace and purity, to bring the best dish of food that existed on earth. Obatalá left and brought back cooked tongue. Olofi was surprised and asked why he brought precisely this dish. Obatalá answered that with the tongue one praises, one says the sweetest and most delicate things, one shows kindness, and one does a lot of good.
>
> The next day Olofi asked Obatalá to bring him the worst dish that existed on earth. Obatalá went away and came back with the same dish as on the previous day: cooked tongue. Olofi was surprised, almost troubled, and said to Obatalá: "Didn't I tell you that I wanted to see the worst food that existed on earth?" Obatalá answered that with the tongue one says the most beautiful things, but with the tongue one also says the ugliest things, bad words, gossip, humiliation, and lies.

With the tongue one can save a person but also cause someone's destruction. And so Olofi was convinced.

Eleggua, the childlike messenger, trickster, and guardian of crossroads, is the most important of the santos in Cuba. He makes communication between humankind and the divine world of santos possible and must always be propitiated at the beginning of every ritual, before the other santos. He is the patron of "all those who do not fit smoothly into or are on the boundaries, in one way or another, of social life" (Curry 1997:68). He opens and closes the doors of people's destinies. Eleggua is known to play tricks with people and can place obstacles in their path; he is therefore deeply respected by everyone. Every Monday he is offered sweets, pastries, and tobacco in order to "open the roads" for his devotees.

In one myth told by a babalao from Havana, the god Olofi suffered from a mysterious and severe illness that made him very weak. All of the santos tried to help him, but their medicines had no effect. Despite his young age, Eleggua prepared a beverage from various herbs. Olofi rapidly became well and decided that Eleggua should always be the first to receive all kinds of offerings. Olofi also gave a key to Eleggua and made him owner of all paths in life.

All humans are said to be related to one of twenty-one varieties of Eleggua. His colors are black and red, and he is represented by a stone or a mass of cement with eyes and mouth made of shells. He has been identified as the Holy Child of the Atocha, although this Catholic name is seldom used. He is placed behind the street door together with Ogún and Ochosi. In this well-known prayer in Lucumí, Eleggua is asked for health and protection: "Owner of the four corners, greatest of the road, my father, take away the bad, so I can walk with much health, so that there will be no illness, so that there will be no loss, so that there will be no revolution, so that there will be no death, in the name of all the children of the house, I say thank you very much, my father Eleggua" (Pérez Medina 1998:326).

Ogún, the santo of war and iron, is the protector of all who are associated with metal, such as blacksmiths, soldiers, chauffeurs, pilots, and policemen. Ogún lends his knife for the performance of sacrifices, and the santero must go through a special ritual associated with this divinity to be allowed to sacrifice four-legged animals. He clears the path for the devotee. He fights for his children and is strong and hard-working. Children of Ogún are therefore often said to be strong, hard-working persons who are never afraid to take on a fight. In one of the myths, Ogún committed incest with his mother. Full of shame he sent himself to work day and night as long as he lived. He is also connected with mountains, agriculture, and the forest, and he knows all the plants. Objects made of iron, such as horseshoes, railway spikes, and miniature hammers and pickaxes, represent him.[1] Ochosi, the divine hunter and ensurer of justice, who is represented by a miniature iron bow and arrow, accompanies him. Prisoners and people who have problems with the law are often said to be his children.

Yemayá is the great mother and the ruler of the seven seas and maternity. She is the mother of many of the other santos, and in one myth she commits incest with her son Shangó. Her colors are blue and white, and she is said to be very understanding, but her character is also compared to the ocean; sometimes calm, sometimes furious. She is compared to the Virgin of Regla, the patroness of the Bay of Havana. When she dances, she imitates the movements of the waves. Her children are said to be harmonious. She controls the reproductive organs and the intestines and is said to be good at healing these parts of the body. One of her representations is that of Olokun, a powerful, androgynous deity who lives at the bottom of the sea. It is common to carry out a ritual dedicated to Olokun to heal all kinds of illnesses and to ensure stability in life.

Shangó, the powerful lord of thunder, lightning, and fire is one of the most popular orishas/santos in Cuba. He is a party-loving womanizer, passionate, and proud of his manly beauty and masculinity. These characteristics make him the idealized Cuban male, and many men claim that they are his children. He is a master of the sacred batá drums, but he is also a fierce warrior with a violent temper who avenges evil deeds. Despite Shangó's masculinity, he may also show himself as the female Catholic saint Santa Barbara, patroness of Spanish artillery.

Oshún owns the river, freshwater, and love. She is also known as Virgen de la Caridad del Cobre, the Catholic patroness of Cuba. A small statue of the Virgin can be found in the church of El Cobre, outside Santiago de Cuba. People from all over Cuba visit the church to pay homage to the Virgin and to be healed from sickness, since she is known to carry out miracles. In the Afro-Cuban myths she is a very beautiful, seductive, sensual, and coquettish santo. She is also passionately in love with Shangó, and in one myth, Shangó fights with Ogún over Oshún's love.

Just as Shangó is the ideal Cuban male, Oshún is the idealized Cuban female. She is the beautiful, independent *mulata* that no man can resist. Her color is yellow, and she is related to gold, honey, and all sweet things. Oshún rules over the genitals and the womb and is called upon in rituals when someone is suffering from a problem with these parts of the body. In one myth she found gold in a calabash. Therefore she is the owner of the calabash, and it is often used in healing related to Oshún. Her children are said to be like her: coquettish, beautiful, and seductive.

The divinity Obba is the legitimate wife of Shangó and said to be very faithful to her husband. She is the symbol of loyalty, but she is of minor importance in Cuba, and it is rare that someone is said to be her child. Oyá, on the other hand, is well known, feared, and respected. She is a warrior and takes part in battles together with Shangó. She is also the owner of lightning and the wind, and the gatekeeper of the cemetery. When someone is very ill, Oyá is asked for help. "If she fails to support him, nothing can be done" (Sandoval 1979:139). Her Catholic names are either Virgen de Candelaria or Santa Teresa.

Osain is the lord of all plants and herbs in the forest. He knows the secrets of the bush and the healing virtues of all herbs *(ewe)* and is often said to be a sorcerer. As he renders healing power to all plants, one must pay him tribute when picking a plant in the forest. According to the mythology, he has no father or mother and has only one arm and one leg, a single eye, an oversized ear that is deaf, and a very tiny ear that hears everything. One myth tells of how he kept the secret of all herbs in a calabash that hung from a tree. Oyá began to swing her skirts, causing a strong wind that knocked down all the herbs. All the santos picked up the herbs and divided them among themselves. They named them and placed ashé in them. Thus, each santo is the owner of a group of herbs, but Osain is still the lord of all of them. He is represented by a small gourd filled with secret herbs and other ingredients, which is often hung from the ceiling in a corner of the house.

The powerful deity San Lazaro, or Babalú Ayé, is also closely related to healing. He is the lord of smallpox, leprosy, skin ailments, infectious diseases, and epidemics and is considered a miraculous healer. He heals all kinds of illnesses but especially those related to the skin. San Lazaro is both highly respected and feared because he may also cause illness. Other names, such as Shaponna, exist for this santo, although they should never be mentioned. It is said that simply pronouncing them out loud might cause illness and epidemics. Among the Yoruba in present-day Nigeria, he is said to be a "hot" divinity associated with hot earth, bad wind, and open spaces "and is the enemy of all aspects of Yoruba urban, corporate culture" (Buckley 1985:128).

His messengers are mosquitoes and flies, carriers of epidemics and illnesses. His body is covered with ulcers, which, according to a popular myth, he contracted because he committed adultery. In another myth, the high god Olofi punished him with syphilis because he lived a promiscuous life with many women (Lachatañeré 1992:270). He walks with difficulty using a crutch, is dressed in sackcloth, and is always accompanied by his dogs, which lick his wounds. Different myths tell of how he brought illness to the world but also how he dedicated himself to healing sick people.

San Lazaro's power to heal is also evident in a prayer commonly offered to him (pronounced in Lucumí): "Father of people and the world, we ask you to give permission in time to express one thing and beg you to give us mercy. We, the believers and your children, know that there exists no other santo as glorious as you from the greatest tradition. Making movement with the wind, taking care of the abundance of illness, dog of illness. Thank you" (Pérez Medina 1998:332).

Orula or Orunmila is another important santo in the santería pantheon. This intellectual deity rules over wisdom and the Ifá oracle, the most extensive and important of the divination systems. Ifá is used by the babalao, the high priest of santería. By divining with the system, the babalao becomes the link to Orula and the high god Olofi. Thus, Orula does not possess humans but communicates through the divination system. He is considered a great "doctor" (Sandoval 1975:156) and is highly respected, and his advice and directives are taken very seriously. He is also known as Saint Francis of Assisi in the Catholic Church, although this name is seldom used.

In the following myth, which warns of the consequences of envy, Orula lives on earth and is a well-known diviner: "Orula walked the earth and everybody was looking for him. He went to a house to divine. When he left, the people in the house broke his divining table and threw away his herbs and his *yefá* (powder). They did this because of envy, in order to hurt him. Orula did not get angry, because his guardian angel had prohibited him from doing so so that he would not lose his luck. After a few days, a man in the house in which Orula had been divining became ill. His relatives went to Orula for help. Orula said: 'I cannot do anything because I don't have anything to work with.' The sick man died."

Ósun is the protector of the initiate. He is always awake, guarding its owner. He is also said to be the head of the initiate and a symbol of the god Olofi. He is represented by an iron bird on a metal staff containing secret herbs and will warn the owner by falling down in case of a serious problem.

Less prominent santos include Inle, doctor of Olofi, a santo related to fishing and hunting who administers and dispenses medicine; Aggayú, lord of volcanoes and the barren plain; Ibeyis, twin children of Oshún and Shangó; Orishaoko, lord of agriculture; Dada, sister of Shangó; Yewa, virgin and santo of the cemetery; and Oddudua/Oddua, a very pure aspect of

Obatalá who gives health and strength of character to those who "receive" him (Díaz Fabelo 1960:63).

Every human being is said to be the child of one or the other of these divinities. As each divinity is related to certain body parts and certain illnesses, it is also often the case that the child of a particular divinity has problems with an illness that a divinity owns or rules over. Accordingly, children of Shangó and Obatalá are more likely to have problems with the eyesight than other people, because these divinities rule over the eyesight. Similarly, a child of Oshún is more likely to have problems with the womb than others.

The santos have great healing powers. Each of them rules over certain parts of the human body, and they can heal the body part or the illness associated with them. But their powers can also cause illness, death, and destruction. An illness may, for example, be interpreted as a call from a santo who wants a person to become initiated and work as a santero or babalao. Initiation is then considered the only way to get rid of the affliction (see also Murphy 1994:87).

If enraged, the santos can punish humans by causing ailments and accidents. Both illness and accidents may be explained by santería followers in terms of punishment for some wrongdoing, such as neglecting the santos. However, more often, the reason for a specific sickness is thought to be a sign from the santo who uses the illness to tell the person that he or she must become initiated and change their life. Often, the part of the body that the santo rules over is affected. Obatalá, for example, rules over the head and the eyesight and may cause blindness and paralysis as a means of "waking up" the person.

Eleggua, who opens and closes roads for man, may affect a person's destiny and open it up to bad influences that can cause illness and death. If he is not propitiated, he may cause "shame, sickness, misfortune and death" (Sandoval 1995:86). Ochosi may send a person to prison. Ogún, who is associated with hard work and iron, punishes by causing problems with the legs and arms and all kinds of accidents that involve iron. He causes trains to derail, while Yemayá, mother of seas, is related to the brain. She can cause drowning accidents, madness, and problems with the intestines.

Oshún rules over the genitals and the womb, and punishes by affecting these body parts and the lower abdomen. As she is the owner of the river, she can also cause drowning in sweet water. Both of these water divinities can also cause tuberculosis through rain and humidity. Oyá, queen of lightning and wind, punishes through accidents caused by strong winds and electricity, and she may cause high blood pressure. Shangó rules over the eyesight and can cause problems with the eyes. He also causes suicides and accidents that involve fire.

Thompson retells one myth of how Shangó himself became the victim of a fire accident as he experimented with a leaf that brought down lightning. His house caught fire and his wife and children were killed: "Half crazed with grief and guilt, Shàngó . . . hanged himself . . . He thus suffered the consequences of playing arrogantly with God's fire, and became lightning itself. . . . He became an eternal moral presence, rumbling in the clouds, outraged by impure human acts, targeting the homes of adulterers, liars, and thieves for destruction" (Thompson 1983:85).

Orula, the intellectual santo and lord of wisdom and divination, punishes by causing madness. He is also consulted through the divination system when a person wants to know if she or he is being punished by a santo. Inle also produces craziness, while Yewa causes tuberculosis using humidity. San Lazaro, lord of infectious diseases, epidemics, and skin diseases, punishes by causing these illnesses as well as gangrene and problems with the bones, but since he controls illness in general he can in fact punish by causing any kind of affliction. One informant told Lewis and his team (Lewis et al. 1978:509) that if someone stole money from the altar of San Lazaro he would punish them by giving them a headache.

Punishment by San Lazaro was also described by the santero Benedí (Lewis et al. 1977a:64): "When somebody gets sores or starts to feel pains, it may be that St. Lazarus [San Lazaro] is punishing him. The only thing the person can do then is pray to St. Lazarus again and again. When he answers and gives his word he'll take the case, then there's no doubt the patient will get well." The relation between the divinities, their colors, and characteristics, and how they punish is summed up in table 1.

Santería, Espiritismo, and the Dead

In santería one always has to pay respect to the spirits of the dead (egún or muertos) before rituals can take place. A ceremony must be carried out in which the spirits are honored. Communication with the deceased is achieved using four coconut shells, the simplest form of divination. The relationship between the santería divinities and the spirits of the dead is expressed in the proverb *El muerto pare al santo* (The dead give birth to the santo).

The idea that people can communicate directly with the dead, deceased family members, or spiritual guides is also present in espiritismo. It is prac-

Table 1. Santería Divinities, Colors, Characteristics, and Punishments

Santo/Orisha	Color	Principle	Divine Punishment
Aggayú	Red and white	Volcanoes, barren plain	Breaking the neck, crushing the body
Eleggua	Red and black	Messenger, trickster, controls destiny	Misfortune, accidents
Inle	Green	Dispenses medicine, fishing, hunting	Madness
Obatalá	White	Peace, patience, purity	Blindness, paralysis
Ochosi	Lavender and black	Hunting, justice	Imprisonment
Ogún	Green and black	Hard work, iron	Problems with limbs, accidents involving iron
Olokun	Blue and white	Profundity	Drowning, madness, respiratory problems
Orula	Green and yellow	Wisdom, divination	Madness
Osain	All colors	Herbs and plants	Madness, nervios, destroying relationships
Oshún	Yellow	Love, beauty, femininity	Problems with genitals and womb, drowning in sweet water
Oyá	All colors	Lightning, cemetery	Accidents with lightning, electricity, and strong wind
San Lazaro/ Babalú Ayé	Purple	Illness, healing	Skin ailments, infections, epidemics
Shangó	Red and white	Thunder, lightning, masculinity	Accidents with fire, problems with eyesight, suicide
Yemayá	Blue and white	Maternity, seven seas	Problems with intestines, drowning, madness
Yewa	Pink	Virginity	Tuberculosis using humidity

ticed by many santeros and has influenced santería. The relationship between the two traditions was summarized by an espiritista: "Espiritismo and santería are like a family; they go together. Before you become a santero it's good to develop your muerto." To "develop the muerto" involves taking part regularly in a spiritist group and becoming possessed until the spirit is under control and begins to express itself in controlled forms.

Espiritismo is frequently present in people's illness stories about santería. Further, it is common that the spirits in espiritismo recommend that a person who suffers from an ailment become involved in santería, and vice versa. One espiritista, for example, explained that he made santo (became initiated into santería) because his muerto told him to do so. According to the muerto, initiation was the only way to get rid of the sickness. The santería divinities, particularly San Lazaro, may also descend and possess the participants during a spiritist mass in order to warn of a serious impending problem, such as an illness or accident.

The spirits of espiritismo may advise a person to carry out a minor santería ritual. During one spiritism session, I witnessed a devotee who was possessed by a spirit recommending that a client put a key in a glass of water and dedicate it to Eleggua, the trickster orisha, messenger of the other santos and lord of crossroads, who opens and closes the roads in the life of a person. The intention here was to open the road for the client. Another muerto asked for sacred water taken from the church of El Cobre, the place where Oshún is represented in the form of the Virgen de la Caridad del Cobre, in order to heal a person.

Rituals

All santería rituals are associated with the concept known as ashé. To be related to the santos means to have ashé (divine power), and humans communicate with the santos in order to get access to ashé. Ashé is "the power to make things happen" (Drewal 1992:xix), it is the source of all power, a "divine current" (Murphy 1993:8) and the ultimate source of everything that refers to balance in the universe (Canizares 1993:5). The santos "feed" on blood from sacrificed animals. When the divinities "eat," ashé is released, and clients are therefore often advised by santería priests to perform sacrifices. If advice is followed and appropriate rituals are carried out, the ashé that emanates from the high god Olodumare-Olofi and the santos will strengthen, protect, and heal humans.

Divination

Three divination systems are used. The simplest and most common is the obí divination that employs four coconut shells that fall in different patterns, with either their concave or convex side up. They answer simple "yes" and "no" questions, such as whether the santos are pleased with a sacrifice. More complex is the dilogún system with sixteen cowrie shells (*C. Monneta. L.* or *C. Annulus. L.*) that fall in different combinations. The santería priests use this system.

The priests keep a number of different sets of cowrie shells as each set is related to a specific santo. To prepare the shells for divining, they are filed down on their backside so that they can fall either on the filed side or with their natural openings upward. If they fall with their natural openings up, it is said that the santo speaks with its "mouth." In order to give the shells strength, they are also washed with omiero and fed with sacrificial blood.

In Ifá, the most complex divination system, a small chain *(ekpuelé)*, usually made of coconut shell or tortoiseshell, is used. On special occasions

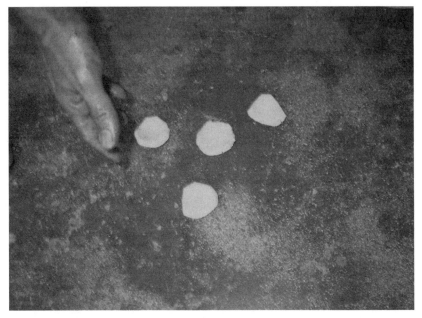

Fig. 11. Obí divination carried out with four pieces of coconut. When all four pieces fall with the white side up, the combination is called Alafi. It is a good sign and means "yes." Photo by Johan Wedel.

when more than one priest is divining, a divination tray (tablero) may be used. The high priest (babalao) who works with the technique is always a man; women cannot be babalaos. He is said to become *maduro* (mature) only after working as a babalao for sixteen years. Divination may produce 256 different combinations. Each combination is related to a large number of proverbs and myths (see Bascom 1980; Matibag 1997). It is therefore impossible for a single babalao to remember them all, even if manuals with some proverbs and myths are in use today.

The Ifá divination system underwent only marginal changes when it was brought from Africa to Cuba. Bascom (1952) has shown how Ifá divination was reinstated "with names and explanatory tales virtually intact" (Thompson 1983:37). In Nigeria, where verses are related to each outcome, a babalao (here called babaláwo) told Drewal in 1986 that nobody had complete knowledge of all the sets of verses: "We still need to discuss it further with other people. . . . Tomorrow somebody might come from Cuba and tell me a meaning of the Olosun meji [his own personal set of verses] and advise me on it" (Drewal 1992:77, brackets in original).

Divination with the coconuts can be learned and used by persons who are not santeros, while dilogún divination can only be used by santeros, and Ifá divination can only be used by babalaos. If someone were to learn and practice the Ifá divination technique without going through the prescribed rituals that make a person a babalao, the outcome would be considered invalid; one must have ashé and the "vibrations" of Orula, lord of Ifá divination, or else the santo will not "respond."

Similarly, one must be a santero or santera, have ashé, and know the right prayers in order to use the dilogún system. When the cowrie shells or the ekpuelé chain are cast in a divination session, each pattern is related to proverbs and to a system of patakíes that involve the santería mythical world and the actions of the santos. Some of the proverbs and myths related to the outcome of the two divination procedures are the same, though there may be considerable variation between the interpretations proffered by different santeros or babalaos.

When someone has a problem, it is common to consult a priest who practices divination, although it has become expensive for people who have to rely on their salary in local- currency pesos. In early 2001, a consultation usually cost twenty pesos (one U.S. dollar) in Matanzas and a little more in Havana. In large parts of Matanzas, and in parts of Havana where there is a strong santería tradition, such as in Regla, Guanabacoa, Marianao, and Habana Vieja, there are a few santeros or babalaos in almost every block.

Many santeros and babalaos make their living by carrying out rituals for clients, from minor sacrifices and ritual cleansing to large initiation cer-emonies, according to the indications of their divination instruments. In order to interpret the outcome of the divination correctly, great skill, experi-ence, and psychological insight are required; the priest interprets the myths and proverbs and relates them to the client's situation and problems (see also Mason 1993). He may also be helped by a muerto who gives informa-tion about the client. During one divination session, for example, the san-tero who had been discussing my relationship to a friend added: ". . . says the gossipmonger who sits next to me." According to the santero, a spirit in the shape of a black woman informed him "in the mind" about clients and their social relations when he performed divination.

Divination indicates whether the problem, such as an illness, is caused by sorcery or by some other agency. Often, the client lacks ashé. When the source of the problem has been established through divination, the priest asks which santo will be responsible for the case and resolve it. Issues con-cerning the client's social relations are often raised in a frank and direct manner as the santero or babalao relates problems to the signs and stories in the dilogún and Ifá divination systems. The diviner often asks the client, "Is it true or false?" or "Am I right?" as he goes on with the interpretation and finally discusses the outcome with the client. In most cases there is little doubt about what to do and what the result will be, if prescribed rituals are carried out in the correct manner. Finally a solution is recommended, usu-ally involving a ritual cleansing (*limpieza* or *despojo*) and some kind of ebbó to one or more of the santos.

Despite the certainty with which the outcome is communicated, the cli-ent may question the priest's interpretation, and in serious cases it is com-mon to visit more than one diviner so as to get an accurate solution to a problem. Uncertainty is part of the divination process, particularly when the problem is said to be caused by sorcery and related to other persons. Sorcery accusations may cause tension and conflict between neighbors, at the place of work, within the family, and so on. In santería, as well as among the Nyole of eastern Uganda, "divination not only attempts to resolve this uncertainty; it also contributes to its maintenance by providing a framework for it. Both uncertainty and its resolution are generated in divination" (Whyte 1997:82).

Today it is common for a santero to perform divination for clients or other persons who may live abroad, even in their absence, and advice about requisite ritual cleansings, sacrifices, or offerings is often given over the phone. Some of these "works" may then be carried out either by the santero or by the client, although this form of divination is believed to be less satis-factory than the one that takes place face to face.

In both the dilogún and the Ifá divinations, as well as in African divination in general, the divination process moves the diviner and the client "out
of their normal modes of thinking, shaking them up in order to change their
minds because their current understanding of the situation is inadequate"
(Peek 1991:205). Two examples of the dilogún divination (an act known
as *registrarse* or *mirarse*) will briefly illustrate the complex process. Before
casting the dilogún shells, the santero prays in Lucumí: *"Omí tutu, ana tuto,
tuto Laroye, tutu ilei"* (Fresh water for refreshing the house, the road [in life],
and for anything that may cause conflicts and problems) (Pérez Medina
1998:109).

The diviner also prays to dead family members and to other related santeros and then says: "There shall be no death, there shall be no illness, there
shall be no tragedy, any bad thing that suddenly arises will move away and
there will be no loss in the family or among godchildren, good things will
come," and then: "Don't say any negative of that which is good, don't say any
positive of that which is bad" (ibid.). The sixteen cowrie shells (in fact there
are eighteen in total, but two are separated from the rest) are cast and the
santero counts how many shells have fallen with their mouths up.

Each outcome (*odu* or *letra*) has a name related to a proverb, which in
turn is related to the myths. If, for example, the cowrie shells fall with three
mouths up, the letra is called Ogundá. The warrior and lord of iron Ogún
speaks in this letra and warns the client of some kind of dispute or tragedy.
Further divination with other divination objects *(ibo)* indicates whether the
outcome is *iré* (positive or good) or if it is *osobo* (negative or bad). In the
negative case the proverb related to Ogundá says, "The knife or the iron
wants war and blood." This means the client is going to have problems with
some dispute that will turn out badly if nothing is done. In one of the
patakíes related to Ogundá, one can find the same message: "A man went
fishing in a place where another person was already fishing. Immediately
when the newcomer threw his bait in the water a fish snatched it. The man
who came first claimed that the fish was his, as it had been swimming
around his bait in order to take it. They began to argue and fight with their
fists. While they were fighting, the fish escaped."

When the santero knows the first sign (letra), he gains some idea of the
client's problem, but he must cast the cowrie shells again to get a more
complete picture. As he continues, the two letras form a combined letra that
also has its own proverbs and myths. The combined letra three-five,
Ogundá-Oshé, for example, reads, "Death is on his feet, problems between
families," and tells of serious conflicts within the family. Another one reads,
"Blood was born through curiosity." If the divination is carried out for a

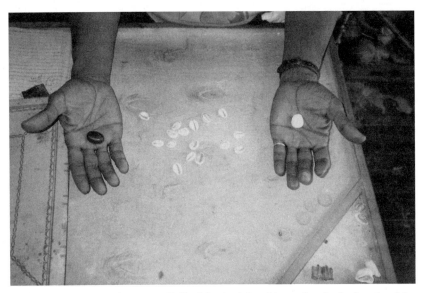

Fig. 12. Divination with cowrie shells, dilogún. The objects, ibo, in the hands of the santero will tell whether the outcome will be positive or good (iré) or negative or bad (osobo). Photo by Johan Wedel.

woman, this particular letra indicates an internal physical disorder and a possible operation. A story related to this proverb tells of how a women was punished by God for her curiosity: she was to bleed every full moon. The santero now has a more complete idea of the problem but continues to divine in order to find out more.

Finally, he discusses the problem with the client and identifies its origin and what has to be done to get rid of or avoid it. He may ask the client about his or her relations with other persons. Often, sorcery is said to be the cause. The priest may recommend some kind of ritual cleansing of bad influences, together with sacrifices, such as killing a rooster and giving the blood to Ogún. He can also suggest that the client receive the protective warriors Eleggua, Ogún, Ochosi, and Ósun. If the problem is very serious the client may be advised to further deepen her or his relation to the divinities and, if indicated through divination, become initiated.

The diviner will not only interpret a temporary situation but also say something about a person's characteristics. If, for example, the cowrie shells first fall with six mouths up, the outcome is called Obara. Each sign has a negative and a positive side, as discussed above. When interpreting the positive aspects of Obara and its proverb "A king does not tell lies," the person is said to be a hard worker, very active and productive, and capable of developing any kind of work to maintain and support self and family. On the negative side, it means the person has daydreams, lives in an unreal world, and is self-deluded.

The person's lack of control over his or her life is here expressed in the saying "Your life is like wheels, they sometimes go up, other times down." The person must learn to shut the mouth, avoid lies, and listen to advice. The shells are cast twice and give, in this example, six-six, Obara Meyi, double Obara. When a double sign appears, it points to a balance between the positive and the negative aspects of the sign but also implies that the person with the double sign easily goes from the extreme positive to the extreme negative side and vice versa. One proverb for the letra six-six says, "The king is dead, the prince is crowned," while another says, "The one who knows doesn't die like the one who doesn't know." A person with this personal letra will have to suffer and work very hard in life, but has good prospects and will always progress.

When the cowrie shells are cast and give more than twelve mouths up, the client is advised to visit a babalao for a more profound reading. The person may be suffering from a serious problem, such as a severe illness, particularly when Metanlá, thirteen mouths, comes up. One of the proverbs for Metanlá says, "Where the illness was born," and the lord of illness, San Lazaro, speaks through the sign. San Lazaro advises the consultant to visit both a babalao and a biomedical doctor for a profound medical examination. It is probable that the person has an illness related to the blood or skin, and it is most likely infectious. The illness may also be a venereal disease, and the person is at risk of having an abnormal child. The client is further advised not to have children with kin, not to mistreat dogs (San Lazaro is related to dogs), and not to curse a pregnant woman, because the curse will affect the fetus. The letra also denotes madness, a fetus that has become the victim of sorcery, and a virgin who has been raped. The general letras in the dilogún system have the following names and proverbs:

0. Oshakuaribo. You are dead but do not know it.
1. Ocanasorde. The world was started by one. If there is nothing good, there is nothing bad.
2. Eyíoco. There is an arrow between brothers.
3. Ogundá. Dispute. Tragedy for some reason.
4. Irosun. No one knows what lies at the bottom of the sea.
5. Oshé. Blood that flows through the veins.
6. Obara. A king does not tell lies. The truth is born from the legend.

7. Oddí. Where the grave was dug for the first time.
8. Eyeúnle. The head carries the body. Only one king can govern a people.
9. Osá. Your best friend is your worst enemy.
10. Ofún. Where the curse was born.
11. Ojuaní. Be distrustful. Water is taken with a hollow basket.
12. Eyilá. Failure for being mischievous. When there is war the soldier does not sleep.
13. Metanlá. Where the illness was born. Bad blood. The one who listens too much to advice will become mad.
14. Merinlá. Envy within the family. Satisfaction if debts are paid.
15. Marunlá. Do not repeat the bad things you did. What moves you, paralyzes you. Dead blood.
16. Meridiloggún. You came to this world to become wise, listen to advice.

The very rare case when all shells fall with their mouth down, *oshakuaribo* (no conversation), implies that the client, or the person who carries out the consultation, will die within hours or minutes. Further divination will reveal the identity of the afflicted. In order to save the person's life, a male goat is sacrificed and its head is buried (Valdés Garriz 1997:100).

Divining the sign of the year

Ifá divination is carried out in a similar way as the dilogún divination. However, Ifá divination is important both for followers of santería and for ordinary people, as is made explicit on the last day of each year. On this occasion, hundreds of babalao priests from all over Cuba and abroad get together to divine *el letra del año* (the sign of the year) "for Cuba and the rest of the world." The priest who has most recently become a babalao will divine, and the most experienced ones then get together to interpret the outcome. The prophecy will guide the spiritual and profane actions of all santeros and babalaos for the coming year. All who have some belief in santería, even if they are not initiated, will also relate to the outcome in certain ways.

When this took place at the end of 1998, about 450 babalaos from Cuba, Spain, Italy, Mexico, Venezuela, Panama, Brazil, Puerto Rico, Costa Rica, Colombia, and the United States gathered in Havana to predict the events of the year 1999. According to the group, the powerful Babalú Ayé, or San Lazaro, the lord of skin diseases and illness, or, to be more precise, an "aspect" of San Lazaro called Azojuano or San Lazaro Misionero, was predicted to rule the year. A series of illnesses such as anemia, leukemia, venereal diseases, and other contagious diseases were predicted to become more frequent during the coming year.

Epidemics would also become more frequent. Violence would increase, hurricanes wreak havoc, and the sea flood the land. It was said that there would be dangers associated with traveling in boats on the sea. Devotees were encouraged to carry out different forms of sacrifice. Among other things, they were told to offer a white chicken, rainwater, and earth from a hill. Everybody, both priests and others, was given advice about measures to be taken, such as making offerings to the sea and being attentive to hygiene and garbage. People were also advised to avoid being disrespectful to their spouses.

When the group met one year later to predict the events of the year 2000, it was said that Shangó would rule the year accompanied by Oshún. Among the illnesses that would increase were disorders related to the heart. There would also be a rise in respiratory disorders and cases of cysts and tumors in the lower part of the belly. The group recommended, among other things, that alcohol consumption be reduced and smoking avoided. Santería priests were told to carry out various works, including making sacrifices and offerings to the divinities and performing a ceremony with calabashes while praying to Shangó and Oshún.

Shangó was also predicted to rule the year 2002, although this time accompanied by Yemayá, queen of the oceans. Among some of the proverbs were the following: "The sheep that associates with a dog eats shit"; "The one who carries fire in his hands cannot wait"; "The one who commits adultery with a man's wife will always be his enemy"; and "A goat that destroys a drum will pay with his skin." The babalaos divined that there would be a rise in cases of thrombosis. There would also be a major increase in deaths related to epidemics and contagious diseases. The group further predicted an increase in wars and breach of contracts, and one or more coups d'état.

People were advised to avoid pork meat, not to store garbage, to avoid violence by any means, and to take care so that children would not go to the beach or river alone. Parents of children born this year were also advised to perform a sacrifice for their children in order to avoid future problems with illnesses and problems related to the blood.

Receiving Santos

Many Cubans have a very diffuse idea of santería and only visit a santería priest when they have some kind of problem, such as an illness. They may carry out a sacrifice or a cleansing ritual, or receive a resguardo (protective talisman), but many do not develop a closer relationship to the santos. If they decide to take the first step into the religion, a *collar* (beaded necklace) is prepared in sacrificial blood. According to Pérez Medina (1998:387), the reason for taking this step may be illness, but it may also be because the santo asked for the ritual during a consultation, or because the person was born with *letra del santo,* born to become initiated. Other reasons given by Pérez Medina are to protect a person from danger, because the person wants to go through the ritual, or because of a spiritual heritage.

The beaded necklaces, according to the combinations of colors they have, represent a certain santo. Like the other objects, these can be bought in many places. The first necklaces a person receives are often the ones of Eleggua (black and red alternating beads) and Obatalá (all white), but others can also be received. In this ritual, the necklaces are washed in omiero, a sacred, herbal mixture made of the plants that correspond to the santo. Sacrificial blood is also poured over the necklaces, and the cotton string that holds the beads together absorbs the blood. By wearing them, the person now wins the protection of the santos.

For the initiate to develop a closer relationship to the santos before going through proper initiation, another important ceremony is carried out: the receiving of Eleggua and the warriors. In order to receive Eleggua, the lord of crossroads, and the warriors Ogún, Ochosi, and Ósun, the first thing that must be done is to acquire the objects that represent these santos. The Eleggua figure is often a stone or a cement head with mouth and eyes made of cowrie shells that the priest who is to carry out the ceremony will make. Miniature iron tools in a small cauldron, which represent Ogún; a miniature bow and arrow that represent Ochosi; and an iron rooster where secret herbs are to be put and that represent Ósun will accompany the Eleggua figure. These objects can be bought in the marketplace, in stores with manufactured goods, or at the yerbero.

In the ceremony, the objects are first received while the person kneels and the priest prays in Lucumí, a creolized form of the Yoruba language, which is used both for recitations and in conversations during rituals. The santero performing the ceremony places the objects that represent his own santos beside the new ones; it is said that the santería objects belonging to the santero "give birth" to the new ones. The objects are then placed behind the main door of the person's house and a rooster is sacrificed. The blood from the fowl is poured over the objects. Eleggua and the warriors will now always work for, defend, and fight for the person. Although these two forms of ritual create a closer relation to the santos, many people never continue beyond this point to go through the proper seven-day initiation.

Initiation

Since the santería initiation costs between eight hundred and a thousand U.S. dollars or more, and an average monthly salary is less than fifteen U.S. dollars (three hundred pesos), people often have to save for years and have good reasons to be initiated. If the person makes the important decision to go through proper initiation, textiles, soup tureens, and other objects corresponding to each of the santos that will be involved in the ritual must be bought. *Otánes* (sacred stones) will be placed in the soup tureens. These stones are usually taken from the seashore or riverbeds and are identified by consulting the obí oracle, the simplest form of divination with four coconut shells. The divination will also reveal which santo is related to which stone.

The otánes not only represent the santos but are regarded as the embodiment of the divinities and will become the most important objects for the initiate. The worship of the stones is explained in a myth in which the high god Olofi gave a forefather eternal life by transforming him into rain. The rain fell down on the earth and turned into a stone. The stone was found and worshipped by his relatives, and it began to work miracles and help humans with their problems.

It has also been established beforehand through divination which santo the person is a child of (although a person's character and behavior will also give some indication), and it is this santo that will be made. The initiate will "give his head" to the santo. According to one santero, this means "the santo will govern you and tell you the good and the bad, past and present." The santo, or guardian angel of the person, will be "put in the head" of the initiate, a procedure called *kariocha*. Things may go badly for the initiate if the wrong santo is made, and to know which santo the initiate is related to is important. Only one santo can be made, and this divinity is called mother or father depending on its gender. It is accompanied by another santo of the opposite gender. If, for example, a person makes Shangó and is accompanied by Oshún, then the father of the initiate will be Shangó and the mother will be Oshún. Other santos are usually also received. They will also protect the initiate but are not as important as the santo that is made.

Some of the divinities, such as Orula, Osain, Olokun, and Aggayú, cannot be made but only received. There are different reasons given for this. Orula communicates by means of divination and therefore does not possess humans. Osain, lord of plants and herbs, cannot be put in the head as "nobody can withstand the forest in the head." Similarly, Olokun cannot be made as "nobody can withstand the ocean depths in the head." Neither can Aggayú because "nobody can withstand the volcano in the head."

Initiation into santería involves a rite of passage (cf. V. Turner 1967, 1969) in which the initiate is reborn and purified and develops a close relationship to a specific santo. The rite of passage is important in santería as it deepens and broadens individual understanding of prior experience and knowledge. It is said that during initiation the person dies and is reborn into the world of the santos, and a very profound and close relationship to a specific santo is created. The initiation generally lasts for seven days, but exceptions exist. If the initiate cannot stay away a whole week, for instance because of their work, the initiation is sometimes shortened to four days.

Liminality, which is the second of the three stages in a rite of passage, has been described by V. Turner (1986:42) as "a fructile chaos, a storehouse of possibilities, . . . a striving after new forms and structures, a gestation process." In santería, the initiate is secluded from the outside world and has to stay in a specially prepared room, cuarto de santo or *igbodu.* Through sacrifices, divination, songs, prayers, music, dance, and possibly possession, the devotee's view of the world begins to change, and a lifelong dependence on the santos is created. After the initiation, the initiate often feels liberated from previous problems, and, if initiation was performed because of an illness, the healing process will begin.

Throughout the ritual an experienced santera or santero, who will become the initiate's godmother or godfather, takes care of the novice and carries out most of the rituals together with the osainista, who is an expert on plants and herbs and their properties, the *italero,* who is an expert on divination, and the oriaté, who directs the ceremonies and knows all the correct words, songs, and prayers to the santos and to the plants and herbs that are used.

Sometimes the same person is responsible for more than one of these tasks. Other santeros will also assist and take part in the ceremonies. The initiation usually takes place in the home of the novice or in the godmother's or godfather's house, *casa-templo.* As the name indicates, the house of the santero is usually both a place of dwelling and a place of worship. The cuarto de santo is where the religious objects are kept and where the most sacred rituals and consultations take place. Less private rituals, such as drumming and dancing, may take place in the living room or on the patio.

Apart from two days when everybody is invited, most of the rituals during initiation are secret, and only santeros are allowed to participate. For some days leading up to the initiation ritual, the main participants refrain from all kinds of sexual activities. On the preparatory day, the iyabó performs offerings in a ceremony called *ebbó de entrada* to ensure that the initiation will be successful. The initiate is first taken to the house where the initiation is to take place, and then to the river where he performs offerings to Oshún. He rips his clothes into shreds and then bathes in the river.

During the first day of the proper initiation, the santo is made. This day is called *el día de la coronacíon* or *asiento* ("seating"), as the initiate is "crowned" with the santo. The first thing to do is to prepare a special kind of herbal mixture and sing to Osain. The procedure is very important because ashé will be released, which, in turn, will bring strength and health to the initiate.

The iyabó also drinks and is bathed with the omiero, which is cool and refreshing and said to contain large quantities of ashé. Omiero is said to be free of violent vibrations (Canizares 1993:102). Similarly, the sacred stones, sacrificial knives, and other objects related to the santos are bathed in the omiero. The santo will be "seated" in the stones, and the santero will then be able to communicate with the stones through divination. The head of the iyabó is shaved and painted in order to invite the santo to come "in the head" of the initiate. A powder made of sacred herbs and other secret ingredients is put on the head of the initiate. The powder is also called ashé, like the divine power that gives life to everything.

Animals are also sacrificed for the particular santo that is to be made. Each santo prefers a specific animal type. To Obatalá, for example, only white animals, such as white goats and white pigeons are offered. The blood from these animals is poured over the sacred stones of the initiate and other sacred objects. Only one santo is made, but usually some of the other popular santos are also received, and blood is also poured over the stones, necklaces, and other objects. During the ceremony, the santeros sing, pray, and ring bells. The initiate is crowned and dressed like a king or queen in colors that correspond to the initiate's santo and is given a new name in Lucumí. The name given is usually related to royalty, such as "king of the people" or "princess of the sea." The initiate is now a child in the process of being reborn.

The following day is "the middle day," when the iyabó sits on a specially made throne and receives visits from other santeros and from family and friends. The visitors kneel and ring a little bell in front of the beautifully dressed and crowned iyabó, and call upon the santo for health and prosperity. I was often told that it was good to tell my wishes at this moment as the iyabó is closely related to the santo and hence to the divine. The meat from the animals that were sacrificed the day before is now eaten.

On the third day (el día del itá), divination with the cowrie shells is carried out with the help of a divination expert called italero. An extended form of the divination procedure that is normally carried out during a consultation now takes place. The interpretations are more extensive and profound. The initiate will be told which camino (road or aspect) of the santo she or he is related to, as each santo has a number of different aspects.

The outcome of the divination tells not only of the initiate's current condition but also of his whole life; the past, the future, his personal characteristics, relations to others, what to avoid, and so on. All sorts of advice is given, particularly regarding food prohibitions, to ensure the initiate a good, happy, and healthy life. If the initiate is a male, he will also be told whether he can become a babalao. The current conditions of persons closely related to the initiate will also be revealed, such as if a husband or child has a serious illness.

The important día de la presentación (day of presentation) is the day when the "newborn" is presented to the three sacred batá drums and a link between the initiate and a particular set of drums is created. The day of presentation is a day of feasting when everybody related to the iyabó comes to honor the newborn and to dance and sing to the drums. During the ceremony, the iyabó and the godmother or godfather, dressed in their royal clothes, dance side by side. Other santeros may also join in. As the music proceeds, the dancers might become possessed by their respective santos.

The ceremony may take place during the seven-day initiation, usually on the fourth day, but may also be carried out at a later occasion. It is a common practice today in Havana for an initiate to carry out the celebration later. Usually a few new initiates get together and hire the drum players for a common ceremony. The reasons for this practice are both that it is expensive to hire the drummers and that there are too few drummers and sacred drums to meet the high demand.

For the two following days the iyabó is kept isolated in the cuarto de santo. Like a newborn child, the initiate is bathed, combed, dressed, and fed. On the last day of the initiation, the iyabó first visits the church. The santería divinities may show themselves in the form of Catholic saints, and the devotee will pay frequent visits to different Catholic churches from now on. The initiate then visits the marketplace where offerings are made. He may also be taken to the jail, to the train station, to the bus station, and to some other places. Presenting the iyabó at all these places ensures that he will not have any problems in the future with justice, trains, bus accidents, and so on. When the iyabó comes home, the soup tureens containing the sacred stones and the other objects are placed in the canastillero.

Life after initiation

The initiation implies a movement from impurity to purity. The initiate is considered pure and newborn after the initiation. If the person is suffering from an illness, a new definition of the ailment is given, which, in turn, is related to the santería cosmology. For one year the initiate has to follow certain rules, will be addressed as iyabó by everyone, and will wear white clothes and a white headdress.

The iyabó is a common sight today all over Cuba and especially in the cities of Havana and Matanzas. The white color signifies that the initiates are under the protection of Obatalá, lord of purity. Initiates may not look in the mirror, they must avoid hospitals, cemeteries, drum ceremonies for the dead, and the coolness of the night, and they may not shake hands with people or stand on street corners. The initiates will also pay respect to other santeros and santería altars by prostrating themselves on a mat. Rules of a more personal nature, revealed in the divination procedure concerning certain obligations and actions, must also be obeyed for the rest of the initiate's life. These personal rules are important in order for the initiate to become healed and to avoid problems.

For the first three months the iyabó must sit on the floor to eat. The ritual called ebbó de tres meses, with animal sacrifices, is then carried out. When the first year is over, a large ceremony including sacrifices, dance, and music also takes place. This day, which is the anniversary of the day the santo was "made," will from then on always be celebrated by the initiate as the "birthday" of the santo. It is the most important day of the year for every santero, and a moment of unification since santeros related to the person, family, and friends all participate.

The devotee has now come under the protection of one of the santos. The santo is called father or mother, and the santero or santera becomes a child of the santo. During subsequent rituals, if the devotee goes into trance and becomes possessed by the santo, the santo is said to be mounting its "horse." These metaphors indicate that the relationship between the santo and the santero is not equal, although there exists an exchange; the santero carries out rituals for the santo, who in turn releases ashé, divine power. But the relationship can never be dominated or completely governed by the santero. This was made explicit during a ceremony when a son of Shangó was sharply told: "You are the slave of Shangó, not the other way around."

The initiate also enters into a life-long relation as a godchild to the madrina or *iyalocha* (godmother), or padrino or *babalocha* (godfather), who was responsible for the initiation. It is said that the initiate becomes part of an *ilé* (a santería household). Further, all godchildren of the same godfather or godmother are called brothers and sisters *(ahijados)*. This quasi-kinship is often said to be stronger than that into which a person is born. The new "family" is important in different ways for all involved as they usually help each other not only with religious matters but with all kinds of problems. Apart from these relations within the family, santería is not hierarchical and has no central authority.

For a practicing santería priest, it is important to have many godchildren not only because of the social support that one may expect, but also because a santero with many godchildren is said to have a great deal of ashé. Initiation also makes the initiate strong and better protected from attacks of sorcery, or, as a santero said: "Sorcery can have a certain effect on me but cannot finish me off completely. My santo is protecting me." Santeros also know how to send back sorcery to its source.

Once the year has passed, the iyabó resumes a normal life and can now decide if she or he wants to learn to become a practicing santera or santero, or a babalao (in the case of men only), if previous divination has not forbidden this. It is possible to become a babalao without making santo. This is, however, uncommon and would mean that the babalao could not participate in all the secret rituals at initiations.

For those who want to work as a santería priest, many years of studying and participation in rituals lie ahead. Much of the knowledge of santería is still transmitted orally and through participation in rituals held by the iyabó's padrino and by others. Because santería's knowledge is immense, it is also written down in notebooks. During initiation, the iyabó receives a *libreta* (notebook) in which the outcome and interpretation of the divination process is written down. The iyabó will then begin to write down ritual practices, prayers, interpretations of divination, plants and their use, and so on. Until recently, the many secret practices, such as certain prayers in Lucumí and the use of plants during initiation, were mainly transmitted orally, but nowadays they can be found in manuals and books (e.g., Garcia Cortéz 1983; Pérez Medina 1998). It remains to be seen if the increased use of written sources will change the forms of teaching and learning santería in Cuba.

Other Important Rituals

The highly secret ceremonies carried out in order to become a babalao are even more elaborate than those used for making santo. Several babalao priests participate, and the divination process is rigorous. A babalao may carry out two kinds of rituals, both related to the lord of divination, Orula. Women who will become godchildren of a babalao receive *cofá de Orula,* while men receive *el mano de Orula.* As with the santero or santera and his or her ahijados, the babalao and the person who carries out these rituals will be closely related. In the case of a male, the mano de Orula ritual may also be the first step on the way to becoming a babalao.

Ceremonies directed to a certain santo are common. A cleansing ritual called *aguán,* related to San Lazaro, is often carried out to heal or prevent an illness. The cleansing can be performed with both initiated and others in the case of serious illness. Another example of a common ritual is the *violín para Oshún* (violin for Oshún). In this ceremony, which is exclusively for Oshún, sweets, cakes, and fruits are offered and the violin is played for the santo. A devotee who has made Oshún may become possessed while laughing in a high-pitched voice and dancing coquettishly to the sound of the violin.

Other examples of rituals are the "food to the earth" ceremony, comida para la tierra, where a sacrifice is made in a hole in the ground. Performed in case of serious illness in order to avoid death, the ritual involves the burial of an animal and other objects instead of the person suffering from the illness. The *ituto* (funeral ceremony), performed to help the spirit of a deceased santero to enter the afterlife of spirits, is later followed by a ritual called *tambor para egún* (drum ceremony for the dead), where a dead santero is honored. Finally, the *pinaldo* is a ceremony related to Ogún in which the right to use the knife for sacrificing large animals is obtained.

All initiates who have made santo have to follow a ritual calendar for the rest of their lives. Every year they will carry out their birthday ceremony, but equally important is the birthday of their godfather or godmother. The ceremony is celebrated by all the godchildren coming together. The santero should also celebrate the annual day of his or her santo; for example, the day of Shangó is December 4, the day of Obatalá is September 24, and the day of San Lazaro is December 17.

During a santero's birthday celebration that I attended, about thirty of the santero's godchildren turned up to help him and to participate in the ceremony, which was to be held over two days. First, a ritual to los muertos was carried out by a small altar on the patio, and divination with four pieces of coconut was used to find out if the dead would give their permission and support the ceremony. It was then time for the santos to "eat," to receive blood, from sacrificed animals.

All the santeros had brought their objects representing Eleggua, Ogún, Ochosi, and Ósun. Eleggua, who mediates between humans and santos, must always eat first or "nothing will happen." An herbal mixture was sprinkled over the objects. A goat was then sacrificed together with various kinds of fowl. The blood from the animals was poured over the objects while the santeros sang in Lucumí.

The soup tureens containing the sacred stones of other santos were then brought forward and a similar procedure was performed. When another four-legged animal, a sheep, was sacrificed, the santero who was celebrating his birthday became possessed with his santo, Shangó. His body trembled furiously, but he soon became calm. His face had changed, and he breathed heavily. He seemed to be looking into another world. With wide-open eyes and nostrils he grabbed a turtle that was to be sacrificed and danced for a short time with it in his mouth. Others became possessed and began to dance. The santero possessed by Shangó celebrated everybody present and advised about health, attacks of sorcery from others, and so on.

A little later the santos left and the possessed became themselves. The meat from the sacrificed animals was finally eaten. As the santero holding the ceremony was the son of Shangó, everybody had a small slice of the fowl dedicated to that santo. By eating the same food as Shangó, the divinity gave the participants part of his ashé.

The following day, santeros, neighbors, family, and friends were invited to a drum feast for the santos, called *bembé*. The ceremony is less sacred than the so-called batá drum ceremony carried out when someone becomes initiated. The drums used during a bembé are less sacred and do not contain the spiritual power found in the batá drums. During this particular bembé, the santero who celebrated was dressed all in red, the royal clothes of Shangó.

Another santera appeared, dressed in a white and blue dress because she was a child of Yemayá. As they became possessed, they danced in front of the drums. A young man suddenly began to tremble and became possessed by Ogún. He was given a piece of cloth related to Ogún and a machete that he swung through the air when he danced.

A woman in her mid-twenties who was standing in the background suddenly began to tremble and swing to and fro. She made a wry face. It seemed as though she was struggling with some kind of force and instinctively we moved away from her. The music was pulling her, demanding her body to move. As she danced, she began to imitate a man shooting arrows. Ochosi, the divine hunter and ensurer of justice, had come down. The ceremony went on for several hours, and people came and went. Finally the drums became silent and the santos left their human hosts.

The woman's possession by Ochosi came as a surprise to everybody because she was not initiated, even though she often took part in drum ceremonies at the santero's house. When I later discussed the matter with some of the santería priests who had been present, they claimed that Ochosi had mounted the woman because he wanted to warn her of a forthcoming problem with the police. The divinity's presence also indicated that she ought to become initiated if she wanted to avoid further problems.

The young woman lived alone with her daughter in a small room with a leaking roof in a run-down neighborhood. In order to improve her situation and earn some money, she was illegally selling souvenirs to tourists. She had been caught twice by the police, and the next time she would be imprisoned, but Ochosi temporarily gave her respite. After the ceremony she decided to become initiated by the santero who had held the ceremony. Within two years she was "crowned" with Ochosi and has not had any further problems.

5

⚹⚹⚹

Healing, Curing, and the Self

Healing in santería is achieved through rituals that include divination, animal sacrifice, offerings, altar building, music, dance, possession trance, and the use of herbs and plants. In this chapter I explore santería notions of self and personhood because these concepts shape the way reality, and illness in particular, are understood within its scheme of thought. I also seek to place these santería notions in a broader comparative perspective. In addressing these questions we gain, I suggest, a deeper understanding of how santería healing works.

Aspects of Santería Ontology

The idea of the self has been widely discussed in anthropology (e.g., Carrithers et al. 1985; Cohen 1994). Here I will use the notion in Willis's (1999:186) sense as "the experiencing human agent" and distinguish it from "the socially constructed" person. In santería, the self is not strictly bound to the individual as in Western cosmology, but may, to some extent, encompass a person's relatives. This is most evident during divination when the santero sees problems and illnesses that belong to relatives of the person for whom the divination is performed. When an illness is sent upon someone through sorcery, this view of seeing other people as extensions of oneself is also apparent; if the intended victim is spiritually strong, someone in the victim's family may instead catch the illness.

When someone becomes initiated, that person will discover his "real self," who he "really is," through divination and will begin to develop a new way of understanding the world. He will form relations to the otherworld of santería divinities, especially to the santo that is "put in the head," to dead ancestors, and to other santeros. He gradually experiences a novel sense of self and begins to see his personal history and future in a new light. Healing in santería is thus, to a large extent, a transformation of the self whereby the initiate begins to experience the world in novel ways. The experience is similar to possession among Tumbuka healers in Malawi (Friedson 1996). In both cases, the devotee will get "access to a wider and deeper world than that of . . . [his] fellow human beings" (28).

The transformation of the self through initiation means that the initiate perceives a protean or expanded self that can also be interpreted as two different selves; the ordinary, everyday self and an emergent "divine" self, a self "made" or "put in the head." This becomes most evident during possession trance when the ordinary self leaves and the divinity takes over. When a santería divinity comes down during possession, the divinity comes to inhabit a person's body temporarily. Through this encounter, humans come in contact with the divine force (ashé), which in turn brings health, luck, and prosperity. To have more than one self is considered pathological in the West (Lock and Scheper-Hughes 1996:54). In santería, possession is considered normal and desirable and is an important part of healing.

A person who practices different religious traditions has a protean self and might become possessed by a number of spirits. A friend of mine, for example, who is well known for his healing skills, is not only a santería priest but also a palo monte priest and an espiritista. Dependent on the context, he may become possessed with the santería divinity Ogún, the palo monte spirit Remolino, his "dead" protector in espiritismo called Francisco, or some other dead ancestor or spiritual guide during a spiritist mass.

In santería ontology, there is, furthermore, no sharp distinction between body and mind. Both during healing and when someone performs sorcery in order to cause an illness or other misfortune, mind and body, self and others are inextricably intertwined. When the initiation ritual is performed to heal a physical ailment, for example, it is said that the person's mental health and social relations will improve as well. The initiate will become calmer and more stable in his social relations, and he will begin to think and feel differently about himself and the world. But he must have faith, or else he will not become healed.

On other occasions, the ritual known as rogación de cabeza is performed to heal mental problems, such as nervios, and give stability in social relations. During the ritual, white objects related to Obatalá, lord of calmness, stability, peace, and purity, are placed on certain parts of the body. Similarly, a sacred herb may both heal a bodily illness and bring peace among family members or neighbors who are arguing and fighting. The use of collares (necklaces) that have been soaked in sacrificial blood and offerings of fruits and cakes are also common to ward off all kinds of illnesses and achieve health.

The interpenetration of self and others is probably most evident when illness is understood in terms of sorcery. When, for instance, a woman suffers from pain in the womb and the problem is said to be caused by someone who has sent illness to her through sorcery, a santero may advise her to change her life and social relations. She may be told to break up her marriage, move to another place, change jobs, or behave differently toward her parents. She may also be told to cleanse her house with herbs against "bad influences," pass a calabash over the lower belly, offer a cake and sacrifice a fowl to Oshún, put on a yellow-beaded necklace, and visit a biomedical doctor.

A further aspect of santería ontology should also be mentioned here: the relation between self and various objects. When sorcery is performed in order to cause a mental or bodily illness, the intended victim's name and his nails, hair, blood, semen, sweat, and urine are often used. In the santería and palo monte view, the person's name, his body liquids, and other things that have left the body spiritually still "belong" to the person and can be used to bring about illness or some other problem. Because of this danger, santeros are generally careful about where they leave and wash their clothes. I was myself advised not to leave my dirty clothes with a washerwoman who was also a santería and palo monte practitioner. If a sweaty shirt were to disappear and then turn up sometime later, I was told I should not use it anymore.

A person may also become mad or invalid by stepping on an object that has been used for spiritual cleansing, or get cancer in a hospital because of a life switch. Further, an evil spirit sent upon someone by an act of sorcery may cause strained social relations and physical or mental illnesses, in both the intended victim and people related to him. Santeros are therefore careful not to step on dead animals, food, and other objects that may be found on street corners, in the cemetery, or in the forest. They are also cautious and observant in hospitals in case of possible life switches.

Santería priests commonly cleanse an afflicted person with an animal so as to "pass over" a physical or mental illness to the animal. In the comida para la tierra ceremony, the animal and other objects that have been used for cleansing are buried and given to the earth to eat in order to prevent the earth from eating the ill person; the animal and the objects are buried instead of the person.

For the santero, this knowledge is important for expelling and preventing illness, but santería healing is more than driving out sorcery and neutralizing evil acts. For the person who becomes initiated, healing is a remaking of the whole world. During the itá divination on the third day of the initiation, the initiate is told through the interpretation of the personal sign or letra how to live his life and what to avoid so as to become and remain healthy, including certain food, certain places, certain situations, and certain people. This reorientation in the world or "alteration of the mode of attention" (Csordas 1994:67) means that the initiate becomes more aware of what may cause illness for her or him in particular. A twenty-five-year-old woman who became initiated because of an illness explained:

> What they [the divinities] take away is what will save you. I was told not to go to the beach and swim in the sea. They took away that. It's because something can happen to me there, like an accident. I cannot eat mutton, colored beans, or *quimbombó* [okra]. I must always wear bright clothes, but I can never wear red. I should not climb up on anything high like a stair, box, or chair because I may fall down. I was told not to keep teeth in the house. I cannot visit a cemetery or a funerary, or carry out any [spiritual] work with people who are dying. If I do that, the spirit may reincarnate in me and take me away.
>
> All this has to do with my health, and all this [the prohibitions] may save me tomorrow. If I have a problem I may be told to give [sacrifice] a sheep to Shangó. That's what he eats. One day I may have to do a cleansing and I take some colored beans and that is what will save me. You go to the santo because you look for health. Not to look for money or anything like that. I did it because of health, and I must fulfill all the rules. If I don't do that something will happen.

For most people, the main reason for initiation is illness, but other aspects of life are also involved, according to a prosperous santero from Matanzas: "Everything will change when you make santo. You exchange illness and death for life, you will have luck and you will progress in order to live well. You will have clothes, shoes, money, a house, women, and children. You will learn new things so you can work tomorrow. If it is an educated man that makes santo, and the santo is made well, the person will be more calm and live a normal life with his wife."

Santería healing and the removal of suffering imply a self-transformation that takes place gradually, sometimes with uncertain outcome. This transformation may begin when a person performs some of the first rituals and receives the beaded necklaces, or receives the trickster divinity Eleggua and the warriors. At this stage, the person may not know much about santería and does not become possessed during rituals. He is just beginning to change perspective and has not yet entered deeply into the religion.

According to devotees' accounts and experiences, deep self-transformation occurs after full initiation. The initiate will begin to move his body in new ways when dancing and praying, and he will possibly become possessed and have an extraordinary experience. Throughout this process, the initiate will be guided by, and be dependent on, his madrina or padrino. Throughout the subsequent year, his or her behavior will be strictly regulated.

Generally speaking, healing is not an event but a process, and santería healing may continue both before and after the seven-day initiation, throughout the whole year after the initiation, and possibly for the rest of the person's life. Although many devotees experience a change and feel healed after the one-week initiation, it is understood that they will fall ill again if they do not live in accordance with their personal divination sign and the advice of the santos. Healing by santería is directed at the whole life beyond a specific healing event.

Encompassing Nature and the Divine

Involvement in santería also means a particular view of the natural environment and a new way of relating to the forces of nature. The santos are closely related to nature, and each of them is considered the owner of a certain group of herbs and plants. According to one of Cabrera's informants, "The santos are more in the forest than in heaven" (Cabrera 1993a:17). The forest is therefore sacred according to santería ideas. In the forest reigns Osain, superior lord of plants and herbs. He heals through his plants that contain ashé.

Each plant species has its mystery, caprice, and even individual psychology that must be known by the person who is about to pick it (117). The forest and the plants must also be paid a tribute before any plant can be removed. By relating to plants as if they were persons, and by participating in an exchange with the forest based on mutual respect, santeros can be assured that the plants will give of their ashé, which, in turn, is necessary for healing and carrying out rituals. If this reciprocity is not acknowledged, the vital force of the plants and the power to heal is lost.

The natural environment is also given a new meaning for the person who becomes initiated into santería, because several of the santos are related to, and considered different aspects of, nature. They own and rule over these aspects. A woman who became initiated two years ago explained: "Before, I respected the sea, but now I respect it much more. It's something indefinite. I made Yemayá, who is the owner of the sea. Since making santo, I don't like to go to the sea, and when I do, I go with a lot of fear and respect. I also think about the herbs in the forest in a different way now. The herbs are alive, and in santería everything is herbs. Many herbs give you stability and power. They have to be respected, and when you cut them, you have to pay them a fee."

Many of the santos are related to the forest, especially Ogún and Ochosi. Yemayá rules over and owns the seven seas, Oshún is the owner of the river, and so on. For the santería devotee, then, the river has both a secular and a sacred meaning. It is both a source of fresh water and the home of the powerful divinity Oshún. Accordingly, the river should be protected and honored because it is related to Oshún. Santería "is based on an understanding that there is no distinction between the natural world of trees, rivers, mountains, and the human world of feelings and ideas. . . . To exist is to have life; nothing is truly dead . . . Man is part of nature. It is his duty to extend and enhance the harmony of his world" (James 1970:40 in Curry 1997:45f).

For the santería priests, it is the river, the sea, and the forest in general that are sacred, not specific named localities, places, or features of the landscape.[1] All rivers are the home of Oshún, and a sacrifice to Oshún may be offered at any of them. Similarly, Yemayá may be honored wherever there is open sea. This redefinition of nature as both divine and part of the human condition also encompasses nonorganic elements. Certain classes of stones, otánes, are considered the embodiment of the santos and therefore living entities. These stones, often found in riverbeds, are the most valued and important objects in santería. During initiation, the stones are asked questions through the divination system. They are also washed in the life-giving herbal mixture omiero and fed with sacrificial blood. Hence, both organic and nonorganic elements of the environment can be considered sacred and possible sources of divine potency.

The santería devotee relates and interacts with the santos through the environment, a relationship that makes the initiate more aware of the environment and gives a broader, deeper, and richer sense of the self. By relating to nature as sacred, the divinities become part of an everyday experience. A santero explained:

> When you make santo you begin to respect nature more. Nature gives life; without it we can't live and we wouldn't be anything. It gives us herbs, animals, everything. In the forest *(el monte)* lives Osain, but also Eleggua, Ogún, Ochosi, Oshún, Aggayú, Shangó, and San Lazaro.

They live in the herbs, they own them. You must ask them to give you permission before you cut them. You have to ask permission from the owner and pray to God, to the earth, and to the sun, moon, and the stars if the herbs are going to have effect.

When someone is ill, you ask and investigate [through divination] which herbs to use. It depends on the illness, and not everybody can use the same herbs. You take them in the morning when they are fresh. It is only when someone has died that you take the herbs in the night to prepare for the *ituto* (funeral). Omiero is made from herbs to drink and bathe with. It is a botanical medicine with great power.

It's the same with the stones, otánes. These are special stones taken from the sea or the river. They are alive. Each of them has an orisha. You have to clean the stone, wash it in omiero, and call the santo in the stone so it will answer your questions [through divination].

Through its relationship to the natural environment and through prayers, dance, music, and possession trance, the self becomes altered and expanded. Through initiation, a lifelong relationship with the otherworld of divinities and spirits is created. The process is similar to those described by Friedson (1996) and Willis (1999). Willis describes it as "the 'self' moving outwards, 'expanding,' the 'spirit' coming in, engaging with the self, entering in and being known" (192). The otherworld is embraced as a source of power to which ordinary, noninitiated people do not have access.

A Note on Yoruba

The structure and ritual elements of the santería initiation have been developed and transformed over a long time but, as mentioned, were originally based on the beliefs of the Yoruba slaves who were brought to Cuba. In relation to the brief discussion of the santería self above, a comparative note on the fourteen-day initiation called Itefa among the Yoruba in present-day Nigeria (Drewal 1992:63ff) is of interest.

The Yoruba ceremonies are performed by the babaláwo priests who use the Nigerian form of Ifá divination. Itefa means "the establishment of the self" and is guidance in life where the diviners not only identify the initiate's personality but also provide him with a set of personal texts that ensure his success in life. The initiation is intended for young boys but may also be performed for adult males who lack "a strong sense of self, . . . and indeed . . . personal wholeness" (72).

In Cuba, initiation is open to both sexes, while in Nigeria only males can be initiated. In both places, though, initiation is considered a rebirth, and the initiate wears white clothes and the head is shaved. The santería initiation, as mentioned, takes place in a specially prepared room called cuarto de santo or igbodu, where the initiate also sleeps when undergoing the ritual. The name igbodu is also used in Nigeria, but here igbodu signifies a sacred grove where the initiate is taken for the first part of the ceremony. In both contexts, sacrifices and dancing are performed.

Similar forms of Ifá and cowrie shell divination can also be found in both places (see Bascom 1969, 1980), and the Ifá divination is an important part of initiation in Nigeria. In Cuba as well as in Nigeria, interpretations of the divination texts serve "as models for self-examination and self-interpretation" (Drewal 1992:63). The aim, both in santería and among the Yoruba in Nigeria, is to develop a strong, new sense of the self that, in turn, is essential when healing illness.

Santería and Biomedicine Compared

There are similarities and fundamental differences between santería healing and biomedical treatment. First, it is important to note that for the person who suffers from an illness, the body is more than a physical object or a physiological state. It is also an essential part of the self and a source of experience (Good 1994:116). In biomedicine, though, the body is often treated in isolation, separated from the mind, and "meaning itself is not configured as a central focus or task" (Kleinman 1995:32). In santería, on the other hand, a bodily illness is related to a larger whole, to social relations, divinities, and spirits.

Another way of looking at this distinction is through the concepts of healing and curing. Healing differs from curing in that healing focuses on meaning and experience in order to "make something whole" that is disrupted or disturbed.[2] Healing "refers to the whole person or the whole body seen as an integrated system with both physical and spiritual components" (Strathern and Stewart 1999:7). Curing, on the other hand, refers to the successful treatment of a specific physical condition, such as a wound or an infection.

Related to healing and curing is the distinction between illness and disease. Illness differs from disease in that illness includes experiences and beliefs. Illness "encompasses the cultural meaning and social relationships experienced by the patient" (Amarasingham Rhodes 1996:171) and "is constituted with an openness to change and to healing" (Good 1994:158). Various illness beliefs can be found in many different cultural settings. Disease, on the other hand, belongs primarily to biomedicine and is specific to Western natural science. Disease is "a biological and biochemical malfunction" (Finkler 1985:5) based on scientific thinking. By these definitions, illness is related to disease as healing is to curing.

Biomedical curing is based on the distinction between body and mind. This so-called Cartesian dualism makes it possible to study and treat the body in isolation, separated from the mind and the social world. The separation, in turn, means that biomedicine often treats illness as either organic or psychological in origin, located either in the body or in the mind, and that biomedicine is reluctant "to range over *all* the domains of Being—personal, social, natural—in diagnostic and therapeutic work" (Jackson 1989:150).

The aims and outcome of healing are also different from those of curing. Healing may aim at a gradual transformation of personal experience of illness, while curing aims at the elimination of a disease or a disorder. Healing depends on satisfaction with treatment, and it is therefore difficult to measure. When patients themselves feel better, "their treatment can be considered successful even if the underlying disease conditions remain largely the same" (Strathern and Stewart 1999:111). Following these distinctions, santería deals mainly with healing and illness. Some santería practices, though, such as when certain plants are used in the cases of diarrhea and no rituals are involved, only aim at curing.

When comparing santería healing and biomedical curing, there is always the risk of the "medicalizing" of religious phenomena, that is, of reducing "the religious meaning of sacred healing to its medical or clinical significance" (Csordas and Kleinman 1996:7; see also Csordas 1987). Santería is a religious tradition often used in order to heal, but to become initiated because of illness is much more than a "treatment." Initiation is aimed at changing the whole life of the individual, a change that is directed both toward the social world and toward a perceived otherworld of divinities and spirits.

Biomedical curing is usually directed only at a certain part of the body, and only the body is treated. But for the person who suffers from an illness, the body is also a part of the self. "The body is subject, the very grounds of subjectivity or experience in the world, . . . a disordered agent of experience" (Good 1994:116). In santería healing, illness is not seen as situated in mind or body alone, since no sharp distinction between mind and body is made. Santería healing is directed toward a transformation of the whole being.

Not all who become involved in santería carry out the seven-day initiation and become santería priests, as discussed earlier. A minor illness may be handled with ritual cleansings or minor offerings, or the receiving of a beaded necklace. In these cases, a major shift in the ill person's perspective and perception of the world may not take place. In all cases, though, divination has to be performed so as to reveal the nature and origin of the illness and the steps to be taken. Consulting a santería diviner and accepting what he says helps clarify the problem and relieve tension and anxiety.

The interpretation is always communicated to the client with great authority because the advice is said to come directly from the santos, not from the santero or babalao. The priests are only vehicles in the transmission of a divine message, and advice is always related to a certain divinity. The diviner emphasizes his inferior position in relation to the santos by saying, "Shangó says . . . " or "Ifá says . . . " or by ending with " . . . says San Lazaro," and says which divinity will be responsible for resolving the problem. This authority may calm down the client. By comparison, a biomedical doctor tends to locate a patient's problem in a certain part of the body in order to give an accurate diagnosis. Often, this is not possible, and the patient is left with great uncertainty about the origin, the treatment, and the outcome of the illness.

For the santería rituals to be successful, the client must have faith. I was often told that if a person does not believe and does not have faith in the santos, he cannot expect anything from them. Another difference between santería and biomedicine is that the patient is almost completely passive when diagnosed and treated by a biomedical doctor, while in santería he or she has to be active. The client must believe and take active part in the offerings, cleansings, and sacrifices prescribed.

Active involvement is also important when santería initiation takes place. Throughout the year after the initiation, the iyabó has to perform certain rituals and follow certain rules and cannot participate in many of the activities of daily life. To obey these rules is to respect the santos. If, on the other hand, the person does not follow the rules, the santos may punish the initiate with an illness or an accident for being disrespectful. A healed person may once again fall ill. The idea of divine punishment is, of course, very different from biomedical explanations of illness.

A santera who now helps others with their illnesses and other problems by performing rituals told me that Yemayá had made her ill because the divinity wanted her to become initiated and practice santería. By making her well through the initiation, Yemayá and the other santos had shown how powerful they were. Through the initiation, the santera was now protected from becoming ill again. The santería view of illness is here very different from the biomedical one: not only is the illness related to the social and spiritual world, but it may also be seen as something positive that can save the person's life.

Biomedicine generally does not recognize that sickness can be socially created. When an organic explanation is found, social aspects and personal histories are deemed irrelevant. The person is seen "as an autonomous unit, independent of and isolated from other individuals and from social and cultural contexts" (Finkler 1994:183). In santería, though, one consequence of initiation is often an improved social life, and the initiate will also develop new social relations with a godmother or godfather, and other godchildren.

It is likely that some of these have become initiated because of a serious illness, and have their own experiences of healing to share with the newly initiated. Santeros often told me that "I know that the santos exist, I have evidence because I was very sick and the santos made me well." This kind of illness experience is important for calming the initiate and convincing him that he will be healed. The biomedical doctor does not usually invoke this kind of personal experience.

The personal experience of the santería priest can be especially important when a client is suffering from a problem that is seen by biomedicine as a psychological illness, such as hearing voices or being possessed by spirits. In the biomedical view, this kind of problem is usually considered to be mental illness. As a result, the afflicted may be treated with chemical drugs. In santería, on the other hand, these experiences are commonly given a religious meaning. The ill person may be told by the santero, who often has his own experiences to rely on, that hearing voices, seeing dead people, and being possessed by spirits are not signs of an illness. These extraordinary encounters with the otherworld are instead interpreted as a spiritual gift that can be used to heal others, as a call from the otherworld, or as an evil spirit that can be taken away or controlled in rituals. The differences between biomedicine and santería are summarized in table 2.

The Coexistence of Santería and Biomedicine

Santería has been important for many people for a long time, although it has been practiced to a large extent in secrecy. Today in Cuba, it is not uncommon that physicians and other health personnel practice, or have some knowledge of, santería. In Havana many physicians are also babalaos, high priests of santería. When santeros and babalaos work as medical doctors, they frequently encourage patients to become involved in santería if religious healing is thought to be a more effective form of treatment than biomedicine. This is especially common when they suspect sorcery, or when they believe that a troublesome spirit is causing the problem.

Table 2. Differences between Biomedicine (Western Medicine) and Santería

Biomedicine	Santería
Directed at curing disease.	Directed at healing illness.
Mind-body distinction. Sickness is either organic or psychological in origin.	No clear distinction between mind and body. No clear distinction between self and others. Illness can be socially created.
Aims at eliminating disease or disorder.	Aims at transforming the experience of illness and self.
Successful treatment may be measured objectively.	Successful "treatment" is related to subjective experience and difficult to measure.
Patient is left with uncertainty when the doctor cannot locate the ailment in the body or decide its origin.	Priest relies on divine power and authority when "diagnosing" the cause of the ailment.
The sick person is passive during treatment and does not have to believe in any external force.	The sick person must be active in rituals and have faith in the divinities in order to become well.
The explanation of sickness is given in biomedical terms.	Divine punishment may result in sickness.
Sickness is a negative experience.	Sickness may be interpreted as a positive experience that can save a person from a bad life situation.
Curing of disease does not change a person's social life and relations.	Santería healing changes a person's social relations and improves social life through initiation.
Doctors do not usually rely on their own sickness experience.	Priests often draw on their own sickness experience.

These interpretations, in turn, are usually given to people who practice santería or some other religious tradition, and often in an enigmatic way. The patient may be told, "This illness may not be of medicine," or "There are other ways." One of the physicians who also works as a babalao is A.M. (see the "life switch" case in ch. 3). He uses medicinal plants and herbs, both as a physician and babalao: "Through working as a babalao I have learned a lot about herbs and plants. If a person is suffering from both a physical and a social problem, I might prescribe an herb that, from a medical point of view, can cure the person. From the religious point of view the plant might also be good for establishing peace and tranquillity in the house or helping the person in his working career by cleansing the way [taking away obstacles]."

Santería priests do not compete with biomedicine. On the contrary, biomedicine is seen as playing an important part when someone is being healed. It is also common to ask the santos through divination if a medical problem has been correctly diagnosed, if a biomedical cure or something else will solve the problem, or if an operation will turn out well. If divination during a santería consultation indicates a health problem, or if a client comes because of some kind of illness, he is always asked if he has seen a physician.

Sometimes a client visits the priest for a minor query but divination points to another, more serious, problem. The sick person is often sent to the family doctor or to a hospital, told to take the prescribed chemical drugs, or advised to change physicians or form of therapy. A babalao explained: "We religious people say that sometimes a person has to attend *el brujo blanco* [the "white sorcerer"] who is the [biomedical] doctor. Sometimes he has to attend *el brujo Yoruba* [the "Yoruba sorcerer"], who is the santero or babalao."

Even if the priest finds out that the problem should be resolved primarily by physicians, some minor rituals are carried out in order to "make the doctors see the problem more clearly." Larger rituals are usually used to facilitate an operation or other more serious medical treatment. If it is established through divination that medical treatment is not sufficient, for example, if the illness is caused by sorcery and is related to the client's social situation, more extensive rituals are carried out. One has to rely more on religious treatment, or, as a babalao who also works as a physician said: "We do this when modern medicine can do no more, when you reach the limit of science." Clients commonly use both santería and biomedicine because one can be "more sure if you attack the illness in two ways, because they make each other stronger. If one fails, the other will resolve it" (Seoane Gallo 1988:4).

In the following case, both santería and biomedicine are used. Lidia, a thirty-four-year-old woman, was initiated into santería because of a serious illness. The ceremony was expensive, but Lidia was lucky to have some relatives abroad who helped her to finance the initiation. When her daughter was initiated into santería three years ago, Lidia was told through divination that she herself had to become initiated as soon as possible. There was a great risk that she could become very ill. She did not take much notice at that time as she felt well. Some months later she went to a medical doctor because she had a lump in one of her breasts. She was told that the lump was nothing to worry about. After a while Lidia went to a babalao, who recommended she change physicians because divination indicated that her problem was serious.

Now she was suddenly told by another physician that the lump was a malignant tumor requiring an urgent operation. This made her very anxious. Her aunt brought her to a santero who confirmed through divination that she had a serious health problem. The outcome of the divination also indicated that she had to be treated by doctors in a hospital but that everything would turn out well if she first performed certain rituals involving sacrifice and then underwent the initiation ritual.

Shortly afterward, she went through the initiation. When I met her a year later she told me that she had been treated at the hospital and also performed the prescribed rituals: "Today I have blind faith in the santos. I feel different today, much stronger and more secure. Before I was very nervous. I was unstable in my relations and didn't have much self-confidence. After the initiation the tumor diminished! I still have to operate to cleanse the breast, but the tumor is totally under control."

The case points to the connection between social relations and individual health and indicates that illness is not considered to be situated in mind or body alone. Lidia's experience also shows how santería and biomedicine are seen as complementary and how santería may interact with biomedicine. Through santería, Lidia is first told to change physicians and then to become initiated, as both santería healing and biomedical treatment are needed. As a rite of passage the initiation also gives her confidence and a new identity. Lidia is now a santera, with a blind faith that the santos are now protecting her from illness. She has developed a new sense of herself and her illness. She feels healthy and, thus, has been healed (though not completely cured).

The episode shows that santería healing may not involve curing; a person can be healed without being cured. Lidia's experience is similar to illness stories of other afflicted persons; it is predicted through divination that the person is or will become ill but at the same time will become healed if certain rituals are carried out. The seven-day initiation becomes an important step giving the initiate a new perspective on life, health, and illness. Through the initiation, a close relation to the world of the santería divinities is created, maintained, and possibly developed further.

The santería priest who initiated and treated Lidia is also a spiritist and practices the religious tradition palo monte. Three days a week he receives people in his home for consultation with the santería cowrie shells. In his story of the event, divination revealed that Lidia had something abnormal in her body, and he saw a forthcoming medical operation.

During the first divination session, the cowrie shells fell in a combination called Metanlá, thirteen mouths up, indicating that Lidia had a serious problem related to the blood and had to expect a forthcoming operation, according to the santero. The lord of illness, San Lazaro, rules over this sign and advice must here be taken very seriously. The client is usually advised to see a babalao for a consultation when a sign exceeding twelve mouths comes up, although it was not done in this case.

The santero also established that Lidia had to carry out a series of rituals and become initiated into santería. A sacrifice (ebbó) to the lord of iron, Ogún, was first carried out. She was cleansed as a cockerel was passed over her body. The fowl was then sacrificed and the blood poured over the sacred objects that represent Ogún. Sometime later she went through initiation and "made," came under protection of, another powerful santo: the lord of lightning and thunder, Shangó.

In the first encounter with Lidia, the santero divined by casting the cowrie shells. First, he got an overall idea of her condition and illness problem. More questions were asked and the shells were cast repeatedly. Her illness was related to, and understood in terms of, the santería cosmology, and Lidia was asked about her problem and her social and personal situation. Finally her problem was clarified as the outcome of the divination procedure was related to the santería proverbs and myths, in this case mainly the mythological actions and adventures of Ogún and Shangó.

Since Ogún is related to everything made of iron, including surgical knives, and particularly the cutting edge of iron (Thompson 1983:52), a sacrifice to him ensured that the operation would turn out well. Sacrifices and cleansing were important here. But since the problem was serious, she was also told to go through the initiation ritual. By asking about Lidia's social relations and by relating the illness to a world of divinities and spirits, her pain and suffering were placed in a wider social, historical, mythological, and spiritual context.

In another case, related by the same priest, a woman in her late forties

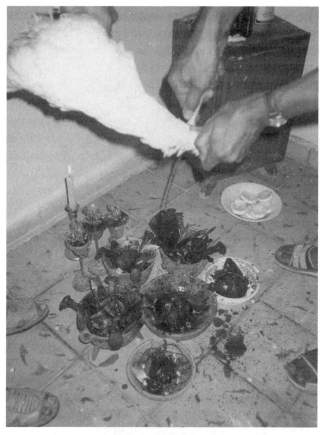

Fig. 13. A fowl being sacrificed for three sets of objects that represent the divinities Eleggua, guardian of crossroads, and the warriors Ogún, Ochosi, and Ósun. Photo by Johan Wedel.

visited a santería priest because she was worried about a sore on her foot. The woman had been to the doctor but did not get better. Divination indicated that she had some kind of problem related to her bones. The priest ordered a bath with herbs. He also put a mixture of crushed herbs on the sore while calling upon the lord of illness, San Lazaro, to help her. When this was completed, the woman was told that she would become well, and she left. Some time passed, then her husband came back to the priest and told him that his wife was not well. Instead she had now been hospitalized because cancer had been found in her foot. According to the doctors, the leg had to be amputated. The priest divined again. Now he found out that the woman had a serious illness related to her blood. The cowrie shells were cast again, and the outcome was interpreted.

The woman could be saved and the leg would not have to be amputated, but only if the woman first carried out a series of rituals to San Lazaro, became initiated into santería, and came under the protection of the divinity Oshún. The sick woman was taken out of the hospital, and she underwent a series of rituals in the forest. Her leg was cleansed and bathed in a mixture of the herbs platanillo de cuba, piñón de botija, and sasafrás, and coco, coconut butter, dry wine, and smoke from a cigar. Animal sacrifices, food offerings, and prayers for San Lazaro were also performed. After a month her leg was fine again; no operation was needed. She became initiated and came under the protection of the santo Oshún. According to the priest, she had to "pay back" and "give her head" to Oshún by becoming initiated because this would protect her from further problems with her leg.

In the illness narrative it is shown how healing is seen as an exchange between the afflicted and the divinity. Oshún will make the woman well and in return is given the woman's head. From the first encounter, both curing and healing are involved. Certain herbs are used for their curative power and put on the sore, but their spiritual properties are also important, and the herbs are applied while calling upon the lord of illness, San Lazaro. In the first encounter with the priest, divination indicated a problem with the bones. Later, this prediction proved to be accurate but the treatment was not initially successful.

On the second encounter, divination revealed that the biomedical diagnosis was not correct; the leg could be saved. The woman could even be healed if a series of rituals was performed, on the condition that she also promised to go through initiation. She was taken to the forest, which pointed to the seriousness of the illness. Here, the woman was close to the healing powers of Osain, lord of plants and herbs. After a month, the sore disappeared and the woman was well. But she would only continue to be well if she went through the initiation and lived in accordance with her santo Oshún. She was healed before the initiation, but only temporarily. The healing was not definite and would only be successful if she developed her relation with the santos, went through the initiation, and followed the advice given to her. This, then, is a case of healing also involving curing.

It is common that santería priests, and occasionally even physicians, advise a person to seek help from espiritismo. The spiritist receives messages from the dead or may become possessed, and many Cubans visit an espiritista when suffering from illness. Often a santería priest who also practices spiritism may use both traditions in consultations, although the respective ritual practices are usually kept distinct in time and space. The physician and babalao from Havana, whom I call A.M., told me that in his work as a physician he is often confronted with possession by spirits:

A.M.: It frequently happens that I have patients who become temporarily absent, their minds become totally empty, and you can't contact them. It is normally interpreted by physicians who do not have any religious knowledge as a hysterical reaction, an absence crisis, or as a form of epilepsy.

J.W.: How are they usually treated by physicians?

A.M.: They are treated with drugs, and it is established that they are mentally ill, or you could say crazy. If neither the patient nor his or her family has any religious knowledge, they accept this interpretation and leave it there.

J.W.: What do you do?

A.M.: If I suspect that it is a spirit, and if the patient's companions have a minimum of religious knowledge, even if it's just Catholicism, I can tell them to take the patient to a place where the person's spirit can be developed. The person might have a spiritual heritage, a spirit that is not necessarily bad, but which lacks clarity and does not leave the person to live in peace.

When the afflicting spirit has been developed over a period of time in spiritual masses, the attacks will be easier to control. The spirit will then normally only "come out" when the medium calls and decides to be possessed. In other cases, though, a spirit is sent through palo monte by an enemy who wants to bring an illness or some other kind of misfortune on its victim. This evil spirit will not be developed but must be taken away.

A forty-two-year-old palo monte priestess from Matanzas, who is also initiated into santería, is often confronted with people who want to hurt someone, but she never obliges. She has a prenda cristiana, an iron cauldron, which is only used for doing good. Many people come to her because they have health problems, and she often advises people to visit a physician: "When a person has a health problem they can come here and ask [the palo monte spirit] if they should visit the doctor, or if the problem can be resolved with palo monte or santería . . . It is common that an illness cannot be resolved with a [biomedical] doctor and therefore people come to my house where it can be taken care of. It also happens that the doctor in the hospital says that you have to look for the occult science, *la sciencia occulta*, because sometimes even the doctor can see that it is a problem that cannot be re-solved with [bio-] medicine."

In sum, santería healing through initiation implies that the initiate will begin to think, act, and feel differently about the self, mind and body, illness, and social relations. In this view, both illness and well-being are closely related to divine and spiritual forces, and nature is given a new and sacred meaning. This view of healing, which often means that illness is related to the sufferer's social world and directed at changing the whole life of the initiate, is very different from biomedical curing. Further, a person may feel healed by santería even if the physical disease condition is almost the same as before.

Santería priests recognize that illness can be socially created. They also emphasize that santería healing means to have faith, to take active part in rituals, to follow divination outcomes, and to visit biomedical doctors. The most striking difference between santería and biomedicine, though, occurs when illness is interpreted as something positive intended to "wake up" the person from a bad life situation: the affliction is seen as both a warning and a chance of a new outlook on life. By seeking the underlying reasons for illness, santería addresses the existential issues that often surround illness.

6

Experiences of Healing

I now turn to an examination of people's experiences of santería healing. Experiences about santería and its ways of healing are often narrated when a group of people are waiting for a divination session or during larger rituals. Santería healing narratives are also common when people discuss illness and healing in general. Listening to the stories may constitute a person's first encounter with santería, and it is likely that they are one reason for santería's remarkable popularity.

The healing narratives recounted here, like all narratives, are partial and subjective, and it is possible that things did not take place exactly as told by the narrators. Nevertheless, the stories have much in common. The narrators experience healing through santería as if they become empowered, strengthened, and protected by the santería divinities. They also acquire a broader view of their illness.

The narratives are all "success stories" told by people who practice santería (and they stand in contrast to the stories in chapter 7 where the opposite view is presented). Apart from the narrators' illness problems, I also briefly discuss the narrators' background, living conditions, and way of life (see also app. 3).

Victims of Sorcery

When I first met Reina, a twenty-eight-year-old Afro-Cuban woman, she had recently returned to Cuba from Europe, where she lives at present. Eight years ago, Reina met a German tourist. After a short time they married and went to live in Germany. They divorced about a year ago, and Reina now lives on her own in a small apartment in a large German city. Over the years, she has returned several times to visit her family in Havana, but this time it was different. Now she had returned because of a supposed sorcery attack that was affecting her both mentally and physically. It all began on Reina's previous visit to Cuba about ten months earlier. A few days before leaving for Germany, she was feeling irritated:

> On the last days in Cuba I felt very uncomfortable. I felt bad and I wanted to fight and destroy all kinds of relationships. I felt terrible. I also had pain in my chest, back, and in my shoulders. It was like a weight that someone had placed over my shoulders. I said to myself that it must be stress, I am feeling stressed because I am leaving. My mother, who is a santera and who has made Yemayá, also felt that something was wrong. She was nervous and asked me all the time if I felt well. She slept badly and woke up all the time. The day before I left, when my mother was cleansing me [spiritually], she began to tremble as if she was becoming mounted [possessed] but nothing happened.
>
> I arrived in Germany and after two days I began to have terrible nightmares. I dreamt that I was trying to close the door to my apartment, but it was impossible because a woman was holding it. The woman, a short mulata with a black skirt and a handkerchief on her head, said: "Don't even try to close the door." The next moment she was holding me very hard in the bed and pushing down my back and shoulders. Then, suddenly, she began to talk in a normal way with me, as a close friend, and asked how I was doing.
>
> I woke up and said: "My God! What is this?" When I fell asleep again, there was another, younger woman who told me she was going to mess with me. She also pushed down my back. I asked her, in the dream, why she was doing this. She told me that "the Chinese" had sent her to finish me off. I don't know any Chinese, and I don't know who she meant. Then the scene changed and it was another woman, this time a black one, who pushed me down. Then another one, then another one.

When the morning came, Reina woke up with severe pain in her back, chest, and shoulders. During the two following nights, she was haunted with the same nightmare, and each morning she felt worse: "I had terrible pain, and it became difficult to get out of bed and even to walk. I became afraid of sleeping, of closing my eyes. I became panicky every time it got dark. I said, 'My God, this is incredible, this pain, I can't stand the pain anymore, I have to call Cuba.'"

Reina's mother was not at home, but her aunt, a renowned espiritista, received the phone call. For her, there was no doubt that it was a sorcery attack. To keep the muertos oscuros at bay, the aunt told Reina to make a cross on the door with pulverized eggshells (cascarilla); to cross all shoes in the bedroom; to place a glass of water under the bed; and to bathe with perfume and cascarilla. "That night I slept wonderfully," she says, but she still suffered the same pain.

When Reina's brother heard the news, he went to a babalao who divined. The priest explained that someone in the family had performed sorcery. This person had sent a dark spirit on Reina with the help of a palo monte priest, and the reason was envy. Reina recalls: "It was someone in the family who was envious of my life, someone close, and it was done with a [palo monte] cauldron. The babalao did not mention any names, but it was a terrible 'work,' designed to kill me. I had pain in my heart and difficulties breathing. The sorcery was carried out in Cuba but with delayed effect. That's why my mother did not feel, or dream, what was going on. Otherwise, her santos would have warned her. The babalao asked my mother how she could miss it, but that was the reason. He said the sorcery was made very well and that they had to act fast to remove it, within ten days."

Reina's aunt held a spiritist session at which a spirit possessed one of the participants and confirmed what the babalao had said; the sorcery had been performed by a close relative, probably a cousin. Reina was in Germany, which meant that the cleansing and removal of the muerto could not be performed on her. The rituals were instead to be performed on her brother because he was "of the same blood" as Reina.

The result would be the same since the santería notion of the self to some extent also encompasses a person's relatives; spiritual works performed on one individual also affect husbands, wives, brothers, sisters, children, and parents. The ceremony took place a few days later. Reina's brother was spiritually cleansed and the bad spirit was removed by sacrificing a pigeon and by using different herbs, cascarilla, liquor, and other ingredients.

Reina remembers that she spoke with her mother on the phone: "I talked to her for a long time. We both cried, and she said, 'I can imagine how you feel, all alone over there.' My mother told me what had happened. The babalao had removed the spirit and placed it in a bottle. When they did the work on my brother, he felt the same pain as I did. For two days, he had a terrible pain in his back, chest, and shoulders, but then it went away. The babalao did the work on my brother and he was affected by the same influence that I had been. We felt the same pain for two days. When his pain went away, mine also disappeared. After that I did not have any more night-mares."

The babalao assured the family that the bad spirit was removed. Reina was nevertheless strongly advised to go through the ritual cofá de Orula and become initiated into santería as soon as she returned to Cuba. The sorcery attack was severe, and the evildoer, or someone else, would probably try again. Reina's brother asked if she could perform some rituals with the santería priests who lived in Germany, but the babalao strongly rejected the idea. He claimed that these santeros could not be trusted for such a delicate matter.

Reina had earlier received the divinities Olokun, Eleggua, and the warriors, which, she says, helped her: "If it wasn't for my santos, which at least gave me some protection, I don't know where I would be today. Many in my family have made santo, and they are [spiritually] protected. Now I also have to do it."

Reina was healed but only temporarily. A few weeks later she began to have the same physical symptoms as before; her chest, back, and shoulders hurt again, although not as much as before. She could live a normal life but was still worried about her pain and decided to visit a physician. He did a short exam and established that the pain was caused by stress. He gave her a prescription for painkillers and a medical certificate, and instructed her to rest for ten days.

Reina followed the doctor's advice but did not improve much, and she continued to feel a vague pain in her back and shoulders. She was not impressed with the medical diagnosis, which was no different from her own first interpretation of her problem. The term "stress" provided no explanation for why this had happened to her and why it took place at that particular time, nor did it account for her terrible nightmares. The interpretation given by the babalao, on the other hand, was profoundly meaningful as it related her suffering to her social world and her present situation.

Reina then returned to Cuba, though, she pointed out, "this time not as a tourist." She explained:

> The first thing I will do now is to give a drum ceremony for Yemayá and then [go through the ceremony] cofá de Orula. I am also saving money to make santo, but that will be the next time I come back to Cuba. I have already bought some cloth, and I will make santo as soon as I can. I don't want to do as my mother did and wait until I am very sick. She almost died in the hospital.

I am still trying to find out who sent the bad spirit. I think it was a cousin who has visited me many times. I saw her in a dream. I am not sure, because my mother's godfather, who is a santero and palero, said it was someone in the neighborhood. I am very confused, but I will continue to investigate this until I know. Now, here in my mother's house there will be sorcery [that is, santería activities] all the time.

In a similar case in which sorcery was "diagnosed," Diana, a woman in her thirties who had access to U.S. dollars and lived a comfortable and prosperous life, was said to have been exposed to evil work that left her partly crippled. Diana could not walk and had problems with her knees. She visited a santería priest for a consultation. Usually the priest would use his seashells as a divination instrument to communicate with the divine world, but this particular time he became possessed with his santo, Yemayá. This is rare, as the santos usually only possess people during large ceremonies.

However, if the problem is serious, as in this particular case, the santos can descend on other occasions: "Yemayá spoke and explained that I had an evil spirit sent upon me. One of my female cousins was to blame as she was envious of my life situation. I work in a tourist hotel and earn some dollars, and that was enough to make her hate me. My cousin had been using hairs from my body by taking them from the soap in the shower. She had gone to a palo monte priest who had an unbaptized cauldron (prenda judía) that is used for evil works. The palero had put my hair and other things in the prenda."

Yemayá also explained what kind of sacrifices and other ritual actions had to be performed and what kind of herbs and plants had to be used to get rid of the sorcery. When the origin of the illness had been established, a series of healing rituals, including animal sacrifices, were carried out. After two months, Diana was apparently walking again. Following the santería and palo monte notion that hair, nails, sweat, and objects that have "belonged to" someone can be manipulated to cause some kind of effect on the person, an evil work had been performed with Diana's hair and personal belongings.

In both Diana's and Reina's narratives, the cause of illness is related to the social world: an envious cousin. They were both exposed to the "dark side of kinship" (Geschiere 1997:11). Illness was understood as originating in sorcery because of envy within the family. The cases also show how a spirit was believed to be involved and how meaning was given to the women's illnesses through santería and palo monte beliefs. In order to heal the two women, ashé had to be restored through sacrifice. Diana did not have to be initiated into santería. For Reina, on the other hand, initiation was necessary to avoid illness and further problems.

Another victim of sorcery is Rosa. She is a beautiful mulata who lives with her parents in a colonial house in one of the residential areas of Havana. Her family was given an apartment in the house when the original owners left after the revolution in 1959. Rosa is about twenty-five years old, and I first met her in the house of her godfather, Julio, who is a babalao. Together with about ten other people, she was waiting for a divination session with Julio. People discussed their problems, illnesses, and experiences of santería. Rosa did not have any profound knowledge of santería but knew many stories of people who had been afflicted by evil spirits and sorcery.

Twice in her life, she says, she has been exposed to sorcery that has resulted in severe illness. The first time, her sister was afflicted. Her sister's body swelled and their mother took her to the hospital. Various analyses were carried out but nothing was found. A doctor then said that if the mother was religious, she should go to a santero because this problem had nothing to do with "modern medicine."

They went to a santero, who concluded that the problem had its origin in sorcery. Evil work had been carried out toward her mother, but her sister had become ill instead as she was spiritually weaker. The santero's interpretation was based on the same notion of the self as in Reina's illness story; the self is not restricted to the individual but also encompasses a person's family. Rosa herself was not afflicted as she has a very powerful spiritual protector: "It was a woman who was jealous of my mother who carried out the sorcery. I did not become ill as my muerto protected me. I can sometimes see him. He is a black man in a white suit and he always smokes a cigar. Well, the santero cleansed us with herbs and other things and our house was also cleansed with herbs. When all this was done my sister became well again."

The second time, Rosa herself became the victim of sorcery and suffered the consequences of an evil spirit a person had sent upon her. Her problems began about two years ago when she felt a severe pain and had heavy vaginal bleeding. She went to the hospital, where it was concluded she had a perforation in her uterus and the uterus should be removed. Rosa's previous experience with sorcery led her to believe that the problem could have a deeper cause.

She wanted to know why this had happened to her: "I saw the perforation with my own eyes when the ultrasound examination was done. I didn't want to remove my womb, and a friend of mine went to a spiritist who said that a muerto oscuro was to blame. It had been sent by someone in order to make me sick and kill me. I was told to pass an egg over my abdomen and throw it outside of the hospital, which I did. I was also told to leave the hospital." Through the act of cleansing, the bad influence was, at least partly, passed over to the egg. Rosa was in the process of becoming healed.

When Rosa left, the flux of blood ceased. The spiritist had told her that she was well protected by her guardian angel Oshún, but she had to consult someone involved in santería in order to take away the evil spirit. She went to Julio, a babalao she knew before, for a consultation. The babalao divined, and Rosa was shocked by the interpretation:

> It was a very bad sign that came up. It was so bad that to speak about it, Julio had to put a silver coin in his mouth. He explained that my problem had its origin in a bad muerto that had been sent on me by my husband's mother, with the help of a palero. Julio told me that my husband's whole family was envious and hated me. I had to carry out a lot of ceremonies. I divorced and left my husband. When I later went back to the hospital for a new examination, the perforation was gone and I didn't have anything! The doctors said it was impossible. They couldn't believe it. Thanks to my padrino [her godfather, Julio] I didn't have to take away anything. Now I come here all the time [to Julio's house].

Julio, the babalao who helped Rosa with her problem, explained:

> The first time she came here it was because everything went bad in her life. She was sick, had pain, and had lost a lot of blood. During the consultation, Orula said she should receive cofá [go through a ritual related to Orula] in order to resolve her problems. She began to come here, and she received Eleggua and the warriors and then cofá. Things became clearer. Orula said her problems were caused by a muerto but that she was not ill, and that she didn't have anything. The doctors saw illness, they saw the perforation, but in reality there wasn't anything. It was the muerto who made them see this. It is also possible it was another dead person's perforation they saw.
>
> It is common that this happens [by acts of sorcery] and the doctors don't understand it is another person they are looking at. This confuses the doctors, who may open up the body and not find anything wrong. Orula also told her to leave her husband's family, as the family only wanted bad things for her. They were very envious of her, as she had a lot of prosperity and luck, and they had used sorcery with paleros so she would not prosper. Before the year had finished she separated

from her husband and left the family. At that time she worked in a hospital but did not like her work. She took a course and got a job in a tourist hotel where her mother also worked. She has seen a change in her life.

This case, which involved espiritismo, palo monte, and santería, also shows how illness is seen as socially created and explained as originating in envy and an act of sorcery; it is related to Rosa's life situation and social world. What looked like a physical illness with a natural cause, vaginal bleeding and a perforation in the uterus, was eventually interpreted as the result of sorcery. The doctors were fooled by the dark spirit sent by her husband's family.

In santería, each sickness that has been caused by a spiritual attack is distinct from any other sickness because every malignant spirit is distinct. Hence, two persons with the same sickness who suffer from a spiritual attack are never treated in the same way. Further, spirits are able both to create a sickness and to create the illusion of it. Some spirits may only produce

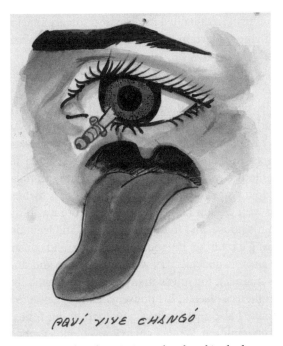

Fig. 14. Handmade painting to be placed in the house to protect against gossip and the evil eye. The text reads: "Here lives Shangó." Artist unknown.

small problems, while others, usually dark spirits, may also cause "real harm" (Seoane Gallo 1988:10f). According to Julio, this would not have happened to Rosa if the doctors had had *videncia* (clear-sightedness) as would have been the case if they had been santería priests or spiritists. When Rosa begins to understand her problem from the santería point of view, her understanding of the illness broadens and produces a change in her whole life situation.

Through santería and its broader view of illness, which often includes magic, mystery, and sorcery, alternative interpretations and possibilities to counter illness are given. The reading of the source of suffering and illness performed by santeros and babalaos gives hope to Reina, Diana, and Rosa. Santería explanations and beliefs help them to imagine and find a solution to their problems (cf. Good 1994:153).

The three women all had access to U.S. dollars and have not suffered the consequences of the economic crisis in the same way as many others. They are among the "winners" in a society that is becoming divided between those who have and those who have not. Their success, however, has nourished feelings of envy among less prosperous relatives, neighbors, and friends. This, in turn, has resulted in supposed sorcery attacks. By entering into santería, divine protection is offered against these malicious deeds.

"I was very bad in my nerves"

Julio, the babalao who helped Rosa, had himself begun to work as a babalao fifteen years earlier as a result of a serious mental problem. After spending some time at a psychiatric hospital, he became initiated and was told that his "way" in life was to divine and work as a babalao. When I met him, he received clients four days a week, from early morning until late afternoon. Sometimes people visited him with motorbikes or cars that had to be spiritually cleansed with certain herbs and leaves. There was always a friendly atmosphere in his house, and many people came and went during the day. Julio was building a room on the roof of his house, and construction workers, who were also his godchildren, were running up and down the stairs. The room was intended for Julio's many godchildren who live abroad. He wanted to offer them a place in his house when they came to Cuba.

In Julio's house I also met Patricia, a woman in her fifties who was another of Julio's godchildren. When I got to know her, I learned that she went to Julio's house almost every day to sweep and clean while he was receiving clients. She divorced many years ago and used to work in a pharmacy but is

now retired and lives alone in a small apartment in a working-class neighborhood in the center of Havana. A few years ago Patricia lost her two sons
almost at the same time. One of them was killed in a car accident and the
other drowned. According to Julio, she saw her dead son in the water and
became almost mad. She received electroconvulsive therapy in a psychiatric
hospital and began to take tranquilizers. When some time had passed, a
friend recommended that she visit Julio for a consultation. She is of African
descent and knew about santería but was not a practitioner. Patricia recalls:

> When I came here [to Julio's house] for the first time I felt very bad
> because I had lost my two sons. I had nervios, I was very bad in my
> nerves, and I was taking pills. I was like crazy and didn't care about
> anything. I was to be taken in at the psychiatric hospital in Mazorra
> [outside of Havana]. I walked the streets every night. Well, I came to
> Julio's house. This was when they turned off the electricity for long
> periods and there were power failures every day, so I kept coming back
> and after a week I finally did the consultation.
>
> I was told everything that had happened [through divination]; what
> had happened to my sons, all the problems I have had, that I had been
> ill, that I felt bad, everything. He [Julio] told me I had to receive cofá de
> Orula. He carried out a sacrifice (ebbó) and a cleansing (limpieza), and
> recommended some [spiritual] baths. I was also told to take some
> [herbal] remedies. The baths were marvelous. I felt so comfortable that
> I began to save money to receive cofá de Orula and went back to Julio.
> [During the ceremony] there came up [through divination] more
> things about my life.
>
> I was told I should never curse or hurt anyone. I was told to receive
> Olokun. I was told what was going to happen in my life and everything
> happened like that. One thing after the other. After that my life began
> to change. My health, money, food, everything changed. I received
> Olokun. The problems with my nerves and my stomach and the pain
> I had in my legs disappeared. I gave up taking my sleeping pills be-
> cause Julio told me I was doing fine. When I went to the doctor the
> third time, he said: "How well you have become, what has happened to
> you?" I told him everything and he himself later on went to Julio for a
> consultation. With love and faith I overcame all my difficulties.

The divination sessions helped Patricia to clarify her situation and to ease
her pain and grief. Her sons' tragic deaths were located in a broader context
and related to other events in her own life. Her life force (ashé) was restored

through sacrifice and she was cleansed from bad, negative thoughts and influences. She received Olokun, the powerful divinity who heals all kinds of illnesses and gives stability in life.

Patricia was healed both by reevaluating her personal history and by being given a new direction in life. She gradually developed a close relation to the spirit world and to the people who frequently visited her godfather's house. Julio guided her on the road to recovery through divinations and rituals. As he himself had suffered from a mental problem, he could draw on his own experience. Helping Julio in his house became important in Patricia's life, and she developed a new view of her self.

Patricia's story is similar to that of Mercedes, a woman in her late fifties, who also experienced nervios and mental problems. Mercedes lives with her son in a small apartment in an old colonial house in a residential area of Havana. During her youth, she was an active member of the Communist Party. Her revolutionary fervor diminished over the years and is today replaced by feelings of disappointment over how the country is run. She is of African descent and claims that her great-grandmother came directly to Cuba as a child, but Mercedes did not have any previous knowledge of Afro-Cuban religions. Twenty years ago she encountered a man whom she had known since childhood. They married and lived happily for a short time, but soon her husband began to suffer from a psychiatric illness:

My husband was bad in his nerves. He didn't want to go out to meet anyone, or to work, or do anything. He hid behind the wardrobe when people came to the house. I was pregnant at the time, and it was really a struggle. Finally, he made santo and began to recover after three months. During his initiation, I was told that I also had to make santo, but I didn't care at the time. I felt well. A few years later I separated from my husband, and sometime afterward I began to have problems with my nervios.

I became really bad. I took poison and pills. I wanted to commit suicide. I didn't even have the force to sweep my own house. I just sat in a chair, and a girl helped me with everything. I thought I was going to die. I even told one doctor I wanted to kill my child and then myself. Six times I was taken in, two of these were at the psychiatric hospital in Mazorra. The doctors said it was a trauma. I was given eight electroshocks in total and a lot of drugs, but I didn't get much better.

When my son later made santo, Oshún descended and said I also had to make santo and that it was very urgent. My ex-husband began to prepare everything, which was not easy because it's very expensive. He was running around to arrange everything and I was bad, bad, bad. My son came home and found me poisoned, and we went to the hospital. There and back, there and back, until I finally made santo.

When I made santo I began to feel a tremendous change in my life. During the seven days in the cuarto I was fed, bathed, and given new clothes. I was like a child who is born. It was quiet. I felt peace and a great tranquillity. During the itá I was given my libreta, and they wrote down which day I was born [became initiated]. They also wrote down the advice of each of the santos. I was told what I had to do and what was going to happen to me. Some of these things have already taken place. I made Caridad del Cobre, Oshún.

The first thing that happened was that I got problems with my legs, which I had been warned about in the itá. I was also told in the itá I had to visit a doctor to check up on my stomach. The santos also told me to take care of my nerves, to always take my medicine, but they said I did not have to receive more electroshocks because I would become well. Sometime after I made santo I felt bad and was taken to the psychiatric hospital again. I also had to go to another hospital because I began to have stomach problems. It was bad because an iyabó is prohibited from visiting hospitals.

The doctors found out that I had chronic gastritis. I left the hospital and some time passed, but I did not get much better and I still had problems with my nerves. There I was with my son and my problems. People said I had been given the wrong santo, and they told me to take off my white clothes. "Why did you do this, you have become worse," they said. I didn't say anything. I thought to myself that I made santo with a lot of faith and that Caridad del Cobre would make me well again. I wanted to be the happy person I was before my illness. My former husband told me I would become well after I made ebbó de tres meses. It was true. I was very thin, but after that I became fatter and I felt better. After nine days I was much better, and people said: "What a change, how well you have become. The santo is great, it makes you believe." They still say that.

I became sick when I was an iyabó because the santo wanted to give me a test in order to see if I really believed. After I made ebbó de tres meses I have not had any problems with my nerves, and I have never been back to the psychiatric hospital. If I feel bad I have my medicines and I put on my collar. I still have my stomach problem, but it is not so bad. When I was ill I cried a lot, but now I laugh, instead. I laugh with a high voice, and people say I laugh like Oshún. When she mounts she comes with a laugh like that. Oshún does not permit me to make santo for anyone else and I don't want to do that anyway. My santos are only for adoration.

I feel very different today. It's like they take away one person and put another in that place. I am not the same as before. I used to be impulsive with a strong character, but now I am more passive and tranquil and I don't argue with anyone. I just laugh because that's my character. Before I used to worry about what to eat tomorrow, but I don't do that anymore. I prepare food for two or three days for me and my son but without the tension I felt before. No, no, that disappeared. My neighbors know my problems and what I went through and therefore they take good care of me. If I get upset, they remind me of how sick I was and tell me that I cannot insult anyone or cause any trouble.

When Mercedes becomes involved in santería, she embarks on a long and difficult journey; her recovery is a gradual process that does not take place in one single event. The divination process clarifies her problems, and she is told how to live her life in the future. Her problems with nervios, as well as her leg and stomach problems, are all related to her personal history. The outcome of the divination and the recommendations she is given also make her more attentive to her problems.

In the initiation room she feels like "a child who is born." After the initiation, while in the liminal and "pure" phase that characterizes the iyabó, she becomes ill again. She has, however, strong faith that Oshún will protect her and make her well. Her illness is now seen as a test of her faith. Mercedes identifies herself with Oshún, the beautiful mulata associated with love, independence, and sweetness. In the process, she becomes more relaxed and less worried about her financial situation. Mercedes is given a new view of her problem and life situation, and she gradually begins to feel healthier. She eventually overcomes her illness, is healed, and never has to visit the psychiatric hospital again. Being protected by Oshún, she will remain healed if she follows the advice received during the divination.

Mercedes's experience with santería is profound; she has developed a new view of herself and not only thinks differently, she also feels different. She is not, however, completely cured as she still takes her medicine and continues to have a slight stomach problem. Her narrative shows how santería healing is used as both a complement and alternative to biomedicine. During the divination procedure that is part of the initiation, Mercedes is told to discontinue electroshock treatment while at the same time taking her prescribed drugs, and to have a physician check her stomach.

In another case, Elena, a twenty-five-year-old woman, also had problems with nervios. Like many young Cubans, she was suffering economic difficulties brought on by the crisis. Elena felt that she had very little control over her own life, and she complained about feeling hopeless, depressed, and dispirited. She did not study or work but just dreamed of winning the lottery held by the U.S. interest office in Havana, where those who won were granted a residence permit in the United States.

At her last job she earned about 130 pesos a month, less than seven dollars. "I spent it in one day and didn't get anything, so why work," she says. When I suggested that she study, she responded: "Yes, but after the studies I might earn at the most four hundred pesos, and who can live on that?" She seldom left the apartment because she "didn't want to see the misery on the street." She related that she had problems with nervios but was also concerned about a physical illness.

Her health slowly deteriorated, and she suffered pain in her lower abdomen. Sometimes she fainted in the street. Elena visited a doctor who told her she had a cyst on her ovary and that it had to grow before they could operate on it. During this time she went to see a santería priest who, through divination, told her that she had to be initiated. Otherwise, she could become very ill and possibly die. She became initiated some months later and came under the protection of the santería divinity Oshún. During the itá, the divination process carried out during initiation, she was told that she had been released from the problems in her abdomen.

Back at the hospital an ultrasound was performed and it confirmed that the cyst had disappeared. Her pain was also gone, together with her depression and nervous problem. Elena told me happily: "From the first day [of the initiation] I felt completely different. I wasn't my old self any more. I felt so full of life. I felt so good, like a little child. When I sat there on the throne I forgot everything. Life as an iyabó is the most beautiful life one can live. I changed completely after the initiation, it was like being born again. Now I feel much more animated. Before I felt dispirited. I had great faith that the cyst would disappear. Faith, together with the santo that you receive [during initiation] and the happiness you feel when you are helped with your health problems, helps you to progress and get rid of your problems."

Despite the fact that her economic situation, which seemed partly to be the reason for her depression, did not change after the initiation, she now has a different view of her own life. She claims that she is protected by Oshún and that she will rely on this santo's powers for the rest of her life.

Elena's story is similar to that of Mercedes in that their suffering was related to the economic crisis. Before the initiation, Mercedes "used to worry about what to eat tomorrow," and Elena felt dispirited because of her difficult economic situation and "the misery on the street." As with Patricia, they suffered from nervios, an ailment that has become common during the crisis and that expresses the hopelessness and powerlessness that many Cubans feel in their lives. Nervios can be seen as an embodied metaphor; it "embodies the lived experience of daily life as a metaphor of physical, social, political, and economic distress" (Low 1994:142).

Nervios is sometimes said to be caused by a troublesome and afflicting spirit. In one case a woman who was considered mentally ill was treated at a psychiatric hospital. She was said to be suffering from problems with nervios caused by a difficult life situation. Some members of her family consulted a santería priest. Divination revealed that the nervous problem had begun because of an evil spirit that she had been afflicted by since childhood and that the divinity Yemayá would help her. She was brought to the priest, who took the evil spirit away and began to heal her. After nine days and several different rituals, she began to feel better. Shortly after, she became initiated and came under the protection of Yemayá. The problems ceased.

Similarly, a woman in her late fifties had spirits that had caused her much suffering for a long time: "About fifteen years ago I had my first encounter with my muertos. I got very sick and thought I was going to die. I heard voices behind me, sometimes telling me what was going to happen. I suffered problems with nervios. At the psychiatrist's I was given a lot of pills and walked around drugged for one and a half years. Finally I met an espiritista who told me to stop seeing the doctor and to develop my spirits. So I joined a spiritist group and participated in their masses. The problems ceased and I began to work with my spirits. Today I receive people with all kinds of problems. Many impotent men come here. I also help women who cannot have children or have problems with their relationship."

These two brief accounts, as well as Patricia's, Mercedes's, and Elena's narratives, suggest that although the explanations of why someone suffers from nervios may vary, it is not until the sufferer becomes involved in santería (or espiritismo) that the ailment is taken care of in a satisfying manner. Through santería, the problem of nervios is reinterpreted and located in life, in a broader context, which includes the social and spiritual world. On the other hand, the narrators' experiences of biomedicine mainly concern the treatment of symptoms with chemical drugs and this, in turn, is perceived as an unsatisfactory therapy. Biomedical practitioners have difficulty treating nervios because it is experienced not in the body but in the world. It cannot be located in a particular site in the body or in the mind. Nervios resists such localization (cf. Good 1994).

A New Outlook on Life

Ana is a woman in her forties. She works in one of the recently opened dollar shops and lives with her son and daughter in a spacious apartment in one of Havana's residential areas. It is a peaceful part of the city with colonial houses, parks, and green alleys. Her mother left Cuba for the United States in 1980 in the so-called Mariel boatlift, when 125,000 people fled the island. After a few years, Ana's mother began sending money, and Ana could finally buy an apartment. Although Ana and her family are of African descent, they did not have any previous experience with santería. Before the family decided to move to Havana, they lived a simple life in a small town in eastern Cuba. A few years ago, Ana divorced her husband. He still visits her, but Ana complains that he is always drunk.

When I first met Ana she was an iyabó. She had recently been initiated and always appeared in her graceful white dress and large white headgear. Three years ago she had very little knowledge of santería and never thought she would become a devotee. She had been suffering from high blood pressure since she gave birth to her daughter about twenty years earlier. She often fainted and had to be taken to the hospital, where she was given injections and different medicines, but the problem always came back. Her blood pressure rose both when she was happy and when she was angry, when she had a soft drink, a beer, a cake, or bread, and in response to many other things.

Ana was worried and visited a santero who divined and told her she had to become initiated in order to get rid of the problem. Sometime later she went through the initiation and made Obatalá, the lord of purity and peace: "During these days everything was so peaceful, a tranquillity that made me feel very good. Everything was done very calmly. I felt very strange, as I was born again. I felt more alert, more vivacious. It was a tremendous experience."

On the day of divination, it was revealed not only that she would become well but also that she had to obey certain rules. For the rest of her life she was not allowed to eat flour, egg, sweet potato, or sheep, or to look at or eat coconut. She was forbidden to get wet in the rain or to expose herself to the sun for long periods: "All this had to do with my health and my blood pressure. I was prohibited from bathing in cold water. When I did that before, I got a lot of pain in my bones. So they [the divinities] took that because it seems that it hurt my bones. I cannot get wet from the rain, either, because the water is also cold and hurts my bones. It's the same with the sun. When I stayed in the sun, I used to get an incredible headache until I could not see. Before I made santo I didn't know why I had such a headache. I thought I had high blood pressure. But it was the sun. That's why they took away the sun."

After the seven-day initiation, Ana had been assured that her problem with high blood pressure was gone. She had a soft drink, "just to try it." The blood pressure did not rise and it has never risen again, she said. The day called "day of the presentation," when she was dancing to the beat of the sacred drums, presented for the drums, was in her case carried out three weeks after the initiation. A lot of people had gathered, and Ana was nervous. Dressed like a queen, she danced in front of the drums and felt something coming down on her: "I felt like I was going to die and I became afraid, I could hear the music very far away. I held on to my godfather, who for a moment told the drummers to stop the music. I cried. It was much worse than when my muerto comes down."

As the drummers restarted, Ana danced again but never went into trance. She says she has not gone to another drum ceremony because she fears what will happen. Ana's experience was profound because she also went through initiation. She has been an espiritista for many years and frequently becomes possessed by her spirit. She often helps people with their health problems in her spiritual "little school" and receives clients who want to develop their spirits. Despite this, the experience with possession by the santería divinities frightened her. During the initiation, Ana calmed down and became aware of what might provoke her illness and pain. Her problem is related to certain situations, and by avoiding these and following the advice given to her during the divination, she is relieved of her high blood pressure problems. She is healed, but only as long as she follows the advice of the santos.

Before the initiation, Ana's whole life situation was affected by her problem. Her illness governed her life and made her worried and anxious. It seemed as if almost anything could make her ill. Feelings, certain foods and drinks, the hot sun, and cold water were sufficient to make her blood pressure rise. She often visited the hospital, where biomedical treatment was directed at lowering her blood pressure with tablets and injections. Her problem was mainly physical, or so it seemed from a biomedical point of view. The healing offered to her by santería, however, was directed not only at her body but also her whole life situation.

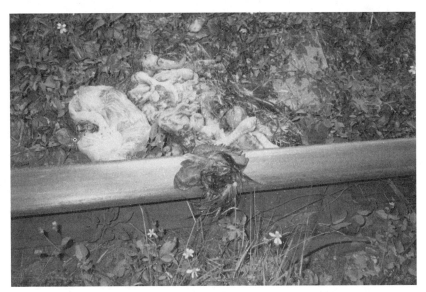

Fig. 15. Sacrifice on a railway line to Ogún, lord of iron. Ogún is said to "live" on the railway line and on the edge of the knife. Photo by Johan Wedel.

During the initiation, she was told how to change her behavior and to live her life if she wanted to become, and stay, healthy. The ritual affected both her body and her mind, and helped her develop a new self. The peaceful experience of seclusion in the initiation room, when she was cared for like a little child, made her feel as if she had been born again. When dancing to the sacred drums, she felt the presence of the divine in her body, but the powerful, giddy experience frightened her.

One of Ana's friends is Silvia. Ana's experience is similar to Silvia's and her husband Mario's encounters with santería and the change it brought about in their lives. They lived in a small and run-down room with a *barbacoa*, an extra floor that they had made for the bed, in the center of Havana, when I spoke to them. They were eager to move to a better place but had not found anything that suited them. "This is not a good place, especially not if we are going to have children. But everything is so expensive," Mario complained. He looked tired and could not hide the fact that some of his teeth were missing. Mario worked in a bakery, and each day he brought home some extra loaves of bread that he sold to friends and neighbors. Silvia used to dance at some of the tourist hotels but had recently become unemployed. "Someone has to stay in the house anyway. If the neighbors find out that there is nobody here, they will break in and steal," she said.

They became santeros with only a little previous knowledge of santería. Their story is typical in many ways of how someone experiences and gradually enters deeper into the religion. Silvia was a mulata, and Mario a Hispanic. Both were about thirty years old. They had met a few years earlier, and neither of them knew very much about Afro-Cuban religious practices. Silvia was twenty-four when she began to have problems with her nerves and pain in her lower abdomen and in her bones. She also had great pain during her menstrual period. A friend took her to a santero who told her, through divination with the cowrie shells, that she had to carry out certain rituals in order to avoid a medical operation. She began to learn about santería.

In her first ritual Silvia received Eleggua and the warriors Ogún, Ochosi, and Ósun, as these santos are always received first and as Eleggua must always be fed with sacrificial blood before any other santo can "eat." Soon afterward, she performed a ceremony and received Olokun, the ruler of the ocean depths and healer of illness. The ceremony included sacrificing a duck and receiving a large soup tureen with shells, sand, and other objects that represent the sea depths. The duck was then filled with seven coins and other objects and given to the sea. During the ceremony Olokun spoke through the divination shells, and the santero who carried out the divination told her to take away the contraceptive she was using, which she did. After three months she felt better in her nerves and the pain in her abdomen was gone, but the pain in her bones continued.

During the rituals Silvia was told that she was born to become a santera and would have to be initiated into santería if she wanted to become well. Five months later she went through the initiation and made Oshún. She recalled the initiation and the year that followed as the most beautiful time in her life: "I felt like a little child. To be a santera is beautiful, but the year as an iyabó is even more beautiful." During the itá (the day of divination), the divination shells spoke about her health, and she was told to strengthen her bones by eating a lot of garlic and different herbs and plants.

She was also told how to get along better with her mother and father; they had been quarreling and fighting for a long time. Shortly after the initiation, their relationship improved and her problems ceased. She claimed that her health has been much better since: "I am always Silvia, but at the same time I feel completely changed. It feels as if I made a life switch. The change has been good and I have a lot of strength and a strong desire to live. Yet, in a way I don't recognize myself. I now have my protective angel [the santo she has made], which is the most important thing."

She was surprised by the respect people showed her during the year that she was an iyabó. Silvia almost never had to stand in line, and everywhere people helped her and let her go first. As a santera she has a different social position in her neighborhood today: "To become a santera is like becoming something big, like graduating from the university. You can feel it from people's reactions. They respect you. When my neighbors' children have fever they bring them to me and I pray to [the saint] San Luis Beltrán for them. Since I have ashé I now also have to help others." When Silvia participates in santería rituals, she frequently becomes possessed by her santo, which, she claims, is a very strange experience:

> When the santo mounts, it first begins with a fit of shivering and a discomfort high up in my stomach. I feel dizzy, like I am going to faint, and I lose balance and coordination. I get confused at first, but I don't lose consciousness. I can still hear everything. Then the confusion is total and I lose consciousness completely and I don't know what is happening. I lose control. It feels as if I am leaving this world. It feels as if my soul is breaking because of pain, similar to when one is suffering. It's never a feeling of anger or rage. Then the santo takes hold of my body completely. This, of course, happens very fast.
>
> Sometimes, I think that the santo will do something shameful and that people will then blame me. After the santo has left, I feel a great spiritual calmness, I feel very pure. All this is like a gift from God and from the santos. It [possession] gives us the possibility to transmit their message.

Silvia's husband Mario was always by her side as she entered into santería. During a divination session, he was told that he also had to become initiated or he would be caught by the police and thrown in jail. At that time he was buying and selling consumer goods and food that were sometimes of an obscure origin. The santo Shangó told him: "You crown me or you go to jail." He decided to become initiated soon afterward.

Before the initiation Mario drank about a bottle of rum a day. Silvia worried about his behavior. She often quarreled with him, saying that he spent the household money on rum, and she complained that he was often drunk. During the divination procedure he was told to stop drinking or he would become very ill and face other serious problems: "When I was one year old I had many epileptic seizures. I was taken to Oyá, to the cemetery, where I went through a life switch, and then I became well. I was told [during the divination] that if I did not stop drinking, the problem would come back." He followed the advice and says that today he feels good: "Now I drink very little and I see things more clearly. I feel better physically and have a strong desire to live. I feel so much love and affection for the santo." Mario was also told that he would one day become a godfather himself with many godchildren.

Both Silvia and Mario stressed that one must follow the directives given during the itá, or everything will go wrong. They also claimed that a santero should do everything with love and attend to the santos and show them respect: "Those who use the religion to become rich will be punished by their own santo."

Silvia's case shows how santería healing includes both pragmatic advice about pain in the body and recommendations about social relations. After the first rituals, the problem with her nerves and the pain in her abdomen were gone, but the pain in her bones was more serious and initiation was required. During the initiation, "the most beautiful time in [her] life," which made her feel "completely changed," she was advised to eat garlic and certain herbs for the pain in her bones. She was also told how to get along better with her parents. After the year as an iyabó, her pain disappeared and her social relations improved. She not only developed a new self; she also became a different person socially. Her neighbors turned to her with their ailments, and she transmitted messages from the santos by becoming possessed during rituals. Silvia thus became spiritually protected and developed a close relation to her santo.

Mario had his own reasons for becoming initiated. He made santo in order to avoid both imprisonment and a forthcoming illness. Through the initiation, Mario became aware of his bad habits and the divine punishment that would follow if he continued to drink and behave irresponsibly. The implicit message was that as long as he followed the advice given to him during initiation, Shangó would protect him.

After their initiations, Silvia and Mario's relationship improved considerably. They quarreled and fought less. Both were eager to become practicing santeros and paid daily visits to their godfather and other santería priests and babalaos in their neighborhood. Occasionally, they brought tourists and other foreigners to their godfather for divination sessions and other rituals. Through the initiation they became part of a new "family" and acquired new social relations.

Silvia claimed that these relations were important for both spiritual and economic reasons: "When a godfather or godchild is sick in the hospital, divination is performed to see what can be done and to make sure that the person doesn't die. There is much sorcery here, and in the hospitals people make life switches. If the person is poor and needs a certain expensive medicine, we get together and buy it."

The dead, muertos, are also frequently said to cause problems because they want the person to change his life. In one of these cases, a forty-year-old man became ill because the muerto wanted him to work as a healer:

> I have had a gastric ulcer since childhood. It became worse and I had to go through several examinations. Later I found out that it was my muerto who was making me sick. It wanted me to work with espiritismo. It took a long time for me to understand that. I am a graduate of the university and I have a certain cultural level. I rejected all that talk about spirits. Finally I started to develop my spirit, but it has taken me a lot of work to change my way of thinking. I don't look for explanations for the things that my muerto does, and I don't question what she says. When she was living at the plane of earth, she was an espiritista. She's Creole and died at the age of ninety-eight.

As he began to "work" with his muerto and to receive other people with illnesses and problems, he began to feel differently about his own illness. The problem diminished: "I still have an ulcer but it has become much better. I feel different and much stronger. I have no pain, I don't feel bad, and I can walk without pain."

In another case, Luis, a retired bus driver, became a babalao a few years earlier because of a serious illness. He is not an Afro-Cuban and did not know anything about Afro-Cuban religions before he became ill. He was fifty-five years old when I met him, and he lived on the ground floor of an old colonial house in a residential area of Havana with his wife and his elderly mother. His house was full of santería objects, and on the floor there was a mat for divination sessions. He was constantly visited by people who wanted him to divine and resolve their problems. Luis retired from his job because he had problems with his back and legs:

> It began seven or eight years ago. Slowly I realized something was wrong as I had difficulties taking a bath and putting on my socks. My joints were losing their flexibility from my waist and down. They became rigid and I began to lose my mobility and the strength in my legs. I also had a terrible pain in my spinal column, so I went to the doctor, a neurosurgeon, who examined me. He told me that I had an illness called arthrosis and that this would continue, that I would lose the sensation in my legs, and that I would become an invalid.
>
> He told me that the solution to my problem was to stretch my spinal cord and that I could be operated upon, but it was very risky and it could easily make it worse. He recommended I leave it there and not

do anything. At that time I had not made santo, but I believed. After a short time, I received Oddua [a very pure and powerful aspect of the divinity Obatalá], and almost immediately I became better. When I left my house I forgot my crutch that I always used, and until today I have not needed it. Nine days later, I made santo. I made Obatalá, which is my guardian angel. During the itá, Obatalá said that this was not the time to go through an operation. He told me to wait six months and then ask Orula. I was also told I was born to become a babalao.

After I made santo I became much better. I was able to walk and even ride a bicycle. The neighbors were very surprised as they had seen how I was before. They said: "Were you not invalid the other day, how is this possible?" The only answer is that I made santo, because the doctors didn't do anything. After six months, I went to a babalao and asked Orula about my situation. Orula said I could have surgery and the santo that would protect me during the operation was Shangó. He also said that everything would turn out fine, but that I had to do a lot of [ritual] work. It was Shangó who told me to go back to the hospital, so I went there with my X-ray plates.

I should have been a lot worse but instead I was much better. I was lucky to meet another neurosurgeon with a lot of experience and asked him if I could be operated upon. He told me that he had to do a lot of analysis but that he would carry out the operation and that I had a very good chance of becoming well. I was so relieved. I went home and continued with my works, and after a short time I underwent the operation. After that I have felt well. My situation changed one hundred percent.

The case illustrates the fact that santería and biomedicine are seen as complementary. Luis relies on both santería and biomedicine in order to resolve his very severe problem. He begins to feel better after first receiving a divinity and becomes even better after the initiation. He has changed, but his problem is not resolved. An operation finally resolves his problem. For Luis, biomedicine is not the only reason that the operation is successful. The positive outcome is dependent on the protection of the santos and the ritual work he has carried out. Because of Shangó's protection and that of the other santos, he is operated upon by the right doctor at the right time and the operation turns out to be a success.

When I made santo I was told I was born to become a babalao. A few years ago I made Ifá [became initiated into the babalao priesthood], and now I help others with their problems. This doesn't mean that I would, for one second, deny the power of science and technological advances.

I have to study all the time. A babalao needs to be studious, but even if we study a whole lifetime it is not possible to memorize and know all the knowledge of Ifá. It contains all knowledge about life. There is not a single life event that cannot be found in Ifá. All of us babalao priests are slaves of Ifá, we have power and knowledge but we have not the power to resolve your problem. No human being has that power. We have the power to tell what Orula is telling. But all the advice Orula gives must be followed or the problem will not be resolved.

Luis did not see any contradiction between santería and biomedicine or, for that matter, between religion and science. They complement each other, although they stand for different kinds of knowledge and meaning. He often sent clients to the hospital or medical doctor, but he also tried to find out the reasons behind afflictions by using his divination system. In addition, he could rely on his own illness experience and recovery through santería. Luis emphasized that he is only a transmitter of divine messages and that it is the client himself who has to be active in order to resolve the problem. Working as a babalao brings him much satisfaction and contentment:

I really like what I am doing. If I had not been a babalao, what would I be doing? I am fifty-five in every sense; physically, sexually, and mentally. What does a poor, retired man, who has passed the age of being useful, do? I would do some errands and then sit on the street corner with the other poor, old people who have nothing to do. Thanks to the religion, I can now work here in my home and do things that result in something wonderful and marvelous.

I can help my mother, my family, and any other person who comes here. Because I am retired I earn 103 pesos a month [about five U.S. dollars], which is nothing, but thanks to the religion we can live well. Often during the ceremonies, when I give the blood [from sacrificed animals] to the santos, we are permitted to eat the meat. This gives us some nourishment. I also earn a little money when I carry out ceremonies, but in my house there is no luxury. I don't have a color TV, but I spent twenty-three thousand pesos when my son made santo. When I made santo I sold my refrigerator, my TV, and other things, and I spent thousands of pesos carrying out my ceremonies.

Of my three sons, two have made santo and the third will do it next year if I have the money. If Orula tells me to carry out some kind of ceremony, I will do it without hesitation. This religion is very expensive, but I am very content. It gives me peace and I live happily. I am a poor man, a fighter, a worker, a starveling. The only richness I have is my honor and the santos that I have been given. They have made me walk and the least I can do is to respect these powers. In this religion we don't speak about what you may gain in Paradise when life is over. This religion includes no concept of Paradise. It helps me, my godchildren, and anyone else who comes to resolve a problem [Luis knocks on the table], in this world where we are living.

Luis is not only healed, his whole life has changed. He is very grateful and now has a close, everyday relation to the santos through his work as a babalao. He has found a new meaning in life as he also helps others in his work. His social situation is different, and he is honored and respected for his knowledge. He is also doing well financially, although most of his money is spent on santería. Luis, as well as Ana, Silvia, and Mario, all felt that initiation into santería led to a considerable improvement in their quality of life. For them, santería healing meant not only recovery from a physical or mental disorder, it also resulted in new social relations, a reevaluation of the nature of suffering, and a new outlook on life.

"There is someone who is protecting me"

Lucia is a thirty-six-year-old woman who lives with her son and daughter in Matanzas. When I first met her, she had been initiated a few months previously and was still an iyabó, dressed in white. She had separated from her husband and her mother had recently died, and she felt depressed. Lucia and her brothers held a spiritual mass for their dead mother. During the mass, the mother's spirit possessed one of the participants and told Lucia to go through the ritual cofá de Orula. The mother's spirit also said that one of her children had to become initiated into santería. Sometime later Lucia went to a babalao and carried out the ritual. During the ceremony, the lord of divination, Orula, told her through Ifá divination that it was Lucia who had to become initiated. Lucia was, or could become, ill and the santo she had to make was Yemayá, the great mother and orisha of saltwater and maternity:

I was very thin after my mother's death, and I was thinking of her all the time. When my uncle became babalao it came up [through divination] that my family as soon as possible had to carry out a spiritual mass for my dead mother. During the mass her spirit came and said that I had to receive cofá de Orula urgently. She also said that one of her children had to do santo because of an illness. My brothers helped me to get the money and within two months I received cofá de Orula.

When I did this, it came up once again that one of us had to do santo and that it was me. I had to do Yemayá. I knew what it meant because many in my family are religious and have santo, but at first I didn't want to do it. I didn't have the courage, and all that money, and one year without going to a party. No. I said to myself that there are people who have not made santo and they are fine.

At the same time I began to feel a small lump in my left breast. I became afraid because my mother had died of cancer in her left breast. I was thinking that now I have to cut off the breast. I didn't want to go to the doctor. I decided to do santo after all, but I didn't know how to get all the money. I don't have a husband, and I make 148 pesos a month. My friends and family said that I was going to be able to do it. Everybody began to help me. A friend of mine who is a santera promised to be my godmother.

Lucia realized she could never afford to pay for the ceremony herself, but her family, friends, and colleagues at her workplace, where she is as a secretary, began to collect money and all the things she needed. Every day people brought her something. Someone brought her cascarilla and candles, someone else a sack of coal. A friend at work even refrained from buying a pair of shoes and instead gave the money to Lucia to buy cloth for the ceremony.

Lucia also borrowed a large sum of money from her godmother to buy the animals needed: "Everybody helped me, and that was the evidence the santo gave me to tell me that I had to become part of my roots. I was born in this, I was raised in this, and the santos were telling me that I could do it. Both my father and my grandmother have made santo. Well, two months later I made santo. My godmother was marvelous. She carried out the ceremony very well and gave me peace in my soul. I made Yemayá and from the first to the last day I felt like a fluid of my mother. She was there."

During the day of divination Lucia learned that she was prohibited for the rest of her life from eating quimbombó (okra), white beans, sheep, and calabash, which she cannot even look at. During the days she spent in the cuarto de santo, the prepared room for the iyabó, Lucia felt very peaceful: "They make you feel like a child, and there are many things that you cannot do. You don't do anything. You are a newborn child in the cuarto, at the foot of the santo. The iyabó cannot shout or talk with a loud voice, or even drink ordinary water. My godmother did everything for me. I was bathed, combed, and she washed my clothes. She gave me food and omiero, which they say makes you strong and fat. I felt like a little child who is discovering new things, like I was born again. It was a marvelous, unique, and unforgettable experience." During the whole seven-day initiation she felt her dead mother by her side. The day of the presentation, when Lucia danced and was presented before the sacred drums, this feeling became even stronger:

> I was so nervous that day, and there were at least twenty people there in the house looking at me. I had a terrible pain in my stomach and had to run to the toilet all the time. When I danced, the nervousness went away. I could feel the spirit of my mother dancing with me and telling me to dance. I forgot there were people around me. I felt alone and I felt that everything I did, I did well. I left, I left in a manner so beautiful I cannot explain it. I know I was there dancing but at the same time I went away. I felt the music in my mind and in my heart, and I saw my mother. It was beautiful, beautiful, something I have never felt before. It was an experience you have to live through in order to understand it. Since making santo I have felt stronger than before, and I am much fatter than I have ever been in my whole life. Before, I used to cry much. I still cry when I think about the fact that I don't have money to pay for this and that, but not as much as before.

After the initiation Lucia went to the hospital, very anxious to investigate the lump in her breast. She had been assured during the initiation that she was now well, but as her mother had died of breast cancer that started with a knot in the breast, she was nervous that her breast would also have to be removed. The physician who attended her suspected a malignant tumor and she was treated directly. Fortunately, it was not malignant. The breast was cleaned and she could go back home. These days she feels good about her life and is happy that she went through the initiation. Lucia says she has been united with her roots because all in her family were followers of santería. She is now well protected by her santo, and her Yemayá is "well put," *bien puesto,* in her head.

Lucia's reason for becoming initiated is twofold. She wants to become protected from illness but also to follow the religious tradition of her family and become "part of [her] roots." The initiation makes her both emotionally and physically stronger. Her experience also points to the importance of spirits of the dead in santería; the spirit of Lucia's dead mother tells her to become involved in santería in order to avoid a serious illness. She is very attached to the memories of her mother and feels her presence: "[The spirit of] my mother gave me an enormous strength. She was herself preparing to make santo when she died."

Two years after my first encounter with Lucia, when the above events were narrated, I met her again. She looked happy and told me that during this time her faith had grown even stronger as she had overcome a serious illness thanks to the help of the santos. The problem with her breast was over. However, recently she had suffered from a problem with her eyesight: "For almost five months I had a great problem with my eyesight because of a blow to my head. I saw very badly, everything was fuzzy, and I had a lot of pain in my eyes and in my head. I went to a doctor but he didn't know how to diagnose my problem, he just said it was something temporary. I could not go to work during this period, and they were almost going to retire me. Well, I also went to my godmother and to my godfather, who is a babalao. He consulted with Orula, and I was given omiero to put on my eyes and to drink. Orula also told me to go back to the doctor, so I went to an eye specialist who began to treat me."

Lucia also participated in a spiritist mass. A spirit called José Lucumí possessed a participant and told Lucia that she would be fine and that he would help her. She also went to a santería drum ceremony where Eleggua descended and told her that he would give his help. Finally she became well. "Thanks to the doctors, God, the santos, my faith, and the [spiritual] work I did, I feel fine today and I'm even working with computers. The santo did his part, he gave me faith to go back to the doctor, and the other part I had to do." As we talked, Lucia stressed how the santos helped and advised not only her but also other people in her surroundings.

When I become sick I become very depressed. But then I go to a tambor [drum ceremony] and a santo descends and tells me, "This is your problem and this is how to resolve it." Then I think, "He will take care of me, there is someone who is protecting me." I become more relaxed, more calm, and I see that the world will not end. This faith even gives me strength to visit the doctor, because when I get depressed I don't want to go to the doctor or anywhere.

The santos give evidence of their existence all the time. First, when you make santo, during the itá, they will tell you which way to take in life. On this road you will find both roses and thorns, but you will triumph. One will always have enemies, santero or not santero, and there will always be people who like you and others who want bad things for you. But if you have your guardian angel [santo] you will be told, through dreams or when you are awake, "Don't do that," or "Do that," or "Don't eat that." During a tambor, a santo may tell me what I should or should not do, and tell me secrets about my life that only I know. This gives me evidence that the santos really exist.

A friend of mine used to have great problems with her asthma. On rainy days she had to rush to the hospital. She made santo five months ago, and her problem is almost gone. She still has asthma, but not the kind of crises she used to have. Another friend of mine was very thin before. She didn't believe in anything but entered the religion because of health problems. Today I can hardly recognize her, she is fat and healthy. It's not the same person. These are signs that the santos give.

Lucia often goes to drum ceremonies but never becomes possessed. When the drums are played, she becomes dizzy and feels a sensation of movement and emptiness in her stomach, which she does not like. During the ceremonies, all the godchildren of her godmother and godfather come together: "It's like I now have a new family with a godmother, godfather, brothers, and sisters. During feasts and initiations we meet. Everybody brings something, like cakes or soft drinks, and when they sacrifice a fowl, for example, you may get a piece of the meat. Everybody works and plucks the fowl and prepares the food. But the help you get is more spiritual than material. We help and advise each other. If I do something wrong they may say, 'Don't do this,' or 'It's like this.' We also give advice to the iyabó, and we say, 'Look, iyabó, it's like this,' or 'This is beautiful, I like it.'"

Lucia's involvement in santería and her encounters with the divine have brought about a new view of the world and a profound change in her life. The possibility of becoming ill with breast cancer does not worry her anymore. She is now on the right road in life. Her santos protect her and give warnings of forthcoming illnesses and other problems.

All the narratives presented here, as well as the stories told by people in the previous chapters, suggest that involvement in santería gives the sufferer a broad view of illness that includes relations both to other humans and to spirits and divinities. In this view, suffering and sickness is not located in either the mind or the body; it is the whole being that is affected. As in the cases presented in chapter 1, the narratives suggest that healing through santería initiation is an open-ended process grounded in bodily experience and directed at a gradual transformation of the self. Problems may be both physical and psychological in origin and are often difficult to treat or define using biomedicine. Some of the narrators also claim that involvement in santería has helped them materially in the struggle against the economic crisis.

The narrators are mainly women. In general, though, men and women practice santería in equal numbers, and when santería divination is performed for clients, men consult santería priests as frequently as women do (see app. 2). Despite this, probably more women than men are initiated, and, during santería ceremonies, women usually outnumber the men. The diviner, on the other hand, is most likely to be a man. The high priest, babalao, is always a man because women cannot become babalao priests.

In many ways the narrators' backgrounds and experiences reflect society at large. Most of them are Afro-Cubans who live, or used to live, in poor neighborhoods. The majority of them also have a working-class background or work in low-income sectors. One must take care, though, not to stretch this generalization too far. Today both Hispanics and Afro-Cubans become initiated. Devotees may be members of the Communist Party, physicians, butchers, scientists, academics, or cleaningwomen. Further, many initiated Afro-Cubans are musicians and athletes who make a considerable amount of money and live in residential areas. Despite this, it is more likely that a santería initiate is an Afro-Cuban who lives in a poor neighborhood with a working-class background. In Cuba, santería ceremonies are much more frequent in poor neighborhoods dominated by Afro-Cubans, such as La Marina in Matanzas or the old parts of Havana, than in the residential areas of Playa in Matanzas or Miramar in Havana.

7

⊗⊗⊗⊗

A Critique of Santería

During the 1960s and 70s, the socialist government and many ordinary Cubans argued that santería was an irrational, unscientific relic of the past that would fade away with development and modern life. Many saw santería as a backward religion that did not belong in the new revolutionary Cuba. In the studies by Lewis, santería was accused by one informant of being criminal, while another referred to it as a thing of the past: "That cult is against science, against modern life in all its aspects. How does being a communist fit in with believing such stuff? It's too great a contradiction" (Lewis et al. 1977a:263).

Among the political leaders it was believed "that popular religions and cult ceremonies would die away with a more educated and scientific approach to life" (Pérez Sarduy and Stubbs 1993:9). A Cuban filmmaker who made a film about the pilgrimage to the Church of San Lazaro in 1961 commented: "I was shocked when I saw them. The contradiction, the superstition. I cannot speak for the new generation and say they will not be religious. I cannot say that they will not believe in God. But I do know that with literacy, in the new Cuba this pilgrimage will not exist" (cited in Brandon 1993:102).

This kind of criticism has today been replaced by critical arguments that focus more on economic issues. Santería priests are now accused of exploiting people financially. The critique, coming from both santería practitioners and nonpractitioners, mainly santería priests themselves and members of various free churches, is often related to the economic crisis and the difficult situation that people experience. In this chapter I give voice both to active santería priests and to people who hold a critical or skeptical stance toward santería.

Today in Cuba, many turn to santería to resolve problems related to the crisis, but the crisis has also affected its practice. A santera from Matanzas told me that santería has now become an expensive religion, only available to those with money: "You have to pay for everything in this religion. You must pay for a consultation, you must pay for herbs and a cleansing. For every procedure you have to pay a fee, and it's expensive." Santería initiations are particularly expensive and often cost more than a thousand dollars. Foreigners who come to Cuba usually pay two to three thousand U.S. dollars. This is less expensive, though, than in the United States, where an initiation may cost six thousand dollars or more (Sandoval 1982 in Matibag 1996:72).

The high costs have meant that some santeros and babalaos who perform larger rituals have become quite wealthy, especially compared to people earning an average monthly salary, which most people find to be ridiculously low. A young woman I met told me that she used to work as a typist in a government office, but her salary was low, about two hundred pesos (ten dollars) a month. When she met a santero, she left her job: "I liked my job, but the salary was nothing. When I met him [the santería priest], he told me that 'the money you earn in one year I can give you in one day.'"

Many complain that people exploit santería in order to get money and that santería priests sometimes recommend expensive rituals that do not need to be carried out. Several people also claimed that santería has become commercialized and that only people with a lot of money can participate. One man who had made santo threw all his religious objects in a river and said that he did not want to have anything to do with the santos anymore "as everything was about money." One santero even blamed writers of santería books and manuals for exploiting priests with a great knowledge of the religion: "Many come here and ask me questions. Then they write books and make a lot of money, but what do I get?" Others argued that some santeros use their knowledge to obtain money from tourists.

According to Luis, a babalao from Havana, the struggle over money may also result in santería rituals not being performed as they should:

Money has changed the principles of this religion. There are people who will do anything for a thousand dollars. They may put Oshún in your head or any other santo, or anything. They exploit santería and give the enemies of this religion justification for saying it is becoming prostituted. Others use fewer things in a ritual than they should, because the animals and everything are very expensive. A priest may

consecrate with less things than are needed. Then there will be problems and failures. A sacrifice is carried out, but you see no result and
people begin to say that they don't have any faith in the santero or in
the babalao.

Another santero from Matanzas also criticized some of his colleagues for
only thinking of money:

Some santeros exploit you. They don't work with faith and love and
with their hearts. If a work costs twenty, they say one hundred. If it
costs one hundred, they say two hundred. If one cigar is needed, they
say five. If you need one chicken, they say five. They do this in order to
satisfy their own needs, to cover their own expenses. They are only
interested in dollars. They want more and more like everybody else,
and without dollars today in this country you cannot clothe yourself,
eat, or anything. They are so interested in the money that they may put
the wrong santo in your head, which can be very bad for you and even
kill you. This has nothing to do with santo, the word signifies someone
who has never committed any sin. These liars will be punished, their
own santo will punish them.

People who suffer from an illness may also criticize and blame santería
for their problems. In one such case, a woman with a stomach ulcer had
been advised, as part of her "treatment," to place a sacrifice in the form of
some fruits and other ingredients in a packet in front of the main church in
Matanzas. This she did. When she left, a man crippled from a muscular
illness followed her: "I knew about this man and I knew people said his
illness was not natural," she said, and continued: "He was really in a bad
condition. He told me that what I had done was a very bad thing. He himself
had once stepped on a 'work' and after that he had become an invalid. He
told me not to practice sorcery and begged me not to leave things in front of
the church. I didn't know what to say and began to cry."

Apart from the supposed victims of different works and the critical santería priests themselves, there are people who have given up their beliefs
and joined other religious groups. They present a powerful critique against
santería, and their stories stand in contrast to many of the other "success
stories." The experience of María is one such example. A few years ago, she
was feeling bad, and a friend took her to a santero. She had pain in her
stomach, worried about everything, and had financial problems. She was
told she would become well if she received the divinity Eleggua and the

warriors Ogún, Ochosi, and Ósun. This she did, but she did not experience any change.

María had the idea that something would suddenly happen in her life if she got involved with santería:

> The only thing that happened to me was that I spent money. I was told I would progress financially and my health would improve, but nothing happened. I spent a lot of money on rituals and offerings, but I never saw any change. I made sacrifice and everything but nothing happened. Finally, I returned everything [the santería objects]. I left the iron things for Ogún in the forest and threw some of the other things in the river. At that time, I lived in a very poor and small room. After some time, I joined the Jehovah's Witnesses and that was when my life began to change. They help me and sometimes I receive clothes. I now live in an apartment, and I feel much better in my soul. God is with me.

Involvement in santería clearly does not always turn out satisfactorily. Neither María's health nor her financial situation improved. For her, santería was more of an investment for a quick return than a gradual development of a new perspective on the world, illness, and self. People who have never become involved in santería and know very little about its practice may also express criticism and skepticism. I met people who found it tragic that santería devotees spent money on rituals and religious paraphernalia despite the fact that, according to the skeptics, they did not have sufficient money to buy food, clothes, and other basic necessities. Skepticism toward santería and other Afro-Cuban religious traditions was especially common among academics and intellectuals, both Hispanics and Afro-Cubans. One university teacher found santería an interesting object of study but claimed it to be an "illusory compensation" for something else.

Others were more neutral and said that they had never had any reason to become involved in, or seek help from, what they labeled as "sorcery," brujería. When I asked a man who was an active member of the Communist Party whether he would seek help from santería if he became sick and the doctors could not cure him, he said: "I don't know anything about santería and I don't believe in it, but yes, if it could help me, I would try it." For many, it is not until they face a serious problem that they become involved in santería and visit a santero: santería becomes the last resort to resolve a problem when everything else fails.

Despite the neutral or skeptical stance from people who do not have any knowledge and interest in santería, it is not uncommon that they have visited a priest for a consultation some time in their life. They may also wear a santería necklace bought in the marketplace. Using a necklace becomes a way of expressing identity and showing belonging to Afro-Cuban traditions, to "follow the roots," even though they remain ignorant of what santería is and how it works. Others, like Ivan, have dedicated many years of their life to the practice of santería.

Exploitation and Manipulation: The Pentecostal Critique

Ivan lives with his wife and three children in a rather poor neighborhood in the center of Havana. He is a Hispanic, and his parents were not familiar with Afro-Cuban religions. During his youth, he began to practice santería and palo monte and continued with that for many years. He lived a prosperous and comfortable life: "I did a lot of illegal business. The santo helped me to obtain what I wanted and I bought everything. But it was dangerous because the police could catch me at any moment and throw me in jail. My children had all the material things they needed, but they didn't have a father. They had someone who was dedicated to other things and did not have time for them."

One day Ivan was exposed to what he calls a "diabolical attack," and his santos turned his luck against him. He was arrested by the police because of his illegal activities and had to pay a huge fine. He lost his money and his car. Ivan began to drink and says that he even wanted to kill himself because he could not give his family all the things he wanted. He was depressed and his wife threatened to divorce him.

> It came to a moment when I didn't wanted to do that [practice santería and palo monte] anymore. I got to know the Word of God. A friend brought me to the Pentecostal Church. I joined them and understood that santeros and paleros are people who manipulate other people. I put all my [santería and palo monte] things in a sack and threw it in the river. Now I am under the protection of the Holy Spirit instead.
>
> People search for tranquillity through santería, but they will never find it. Instead, they will be manipulated. One day you have to put on a necklace, the next day sacrifice a chicken, the next day a sheep, and finally you have to make santo. Here in Cuba we are still victims of this manipulation and slavery. The santero may resolve a problem for you. Then you come back and are very grateful. But then something else

happens that gives you a new problem, and you have to go back and resolve that too, and invest more money. The santero will make you dependent on him and his santos.

During a consultation it's possible that the santero will tell you that you have a muerto oscuro behind you and that you will have a lot of problems. He will then offer himself to help you and take the spirit away, and you have to pay more and more. People are capable of selling their refrigerators, TV sets, and beds, and spending all their money on making santo in order to try to change their lives. Today, a lot of foreigners come here to make santo because it costs less than in other countries. But they are also exploited and have to pay three, four, or five thousand dollars. It works like this: I have santería business and ask you, as a foreigner, to bring me other foreigners to make santo. Then we split the money between us.

Ivan still believes that the santos can punish people and that magic may have an effect. At the same time he is very skeptical about santería's power to resolve problems and heal illness. Instead, he claims, it makes people suffer even more.

If you leave santería and don't want to participate anymore, and you are without any protection from God and the Holy Spirit, it can be very dangerous. You can be punished by the santos or by your godfather. The santero has a certain power over his godchildren. He can make them come to him through different works. He will use fire or "bind" them and, for example, destroy a marriage so that the godchild will come back to him.

If you go to El Rincón and the Church of San Lazaro in December, you will see people who walk for kilometers on their bloody knees in order to save an ill family member. What kind of religion is that that makes people suffer like that? It's not right, and nobody needs to use a necklace or sacrifice an animal in order to resolve a problem.

When someone makes santo because of illness, that person may become well for a short time but then everything will be the same as before. It's better to go to the [Pentecostal] church. In every [Pentecostal] church there are people who have been healed from illnesses that science couldn't do anything about.

Teresa is about fifty years old and also a member of the Pentecostal Church. She lives in a modern apartment in a working-class neighborhood in the center of Havana with her daughter, son-in-law, and their only child.

The living room has little furniture. A Bible and the texts of some religious songs are on the sofa. In one corner stands an organ and on the wall hang a homemade crucifix and posters from the Pentecostal Church. Teresa, who is an Afro-Cuban, grew up with parents practicing both santería and palo monte. For more than thirty years, she was a very active santera, palera, and espiritista. Some of her neighbors even called her a fanatic. She was a daughter of Yemayá and a well-known diviner. She had many godchildren, did all kinds of work, and was consulted by both Cubans and foreigners. "I healed people," she says.

Once, she carried out a life switch (cambio de vida), in order to save a young girl's life:

> A friend of mine gave birth to a child who was very ill. The whole family was at the hospital, crying. I said: "We will save the child and bring her out of the hospital." The child could die at any moment. I had brought a doll that was prepared with smoke from a cigar, corn, beans, rice, sugar, salt, candles, *aguardiente* [spirituous liquor], cascarilla, and herbs like rompezaragüey, vencedor, abrecamino, and muralla. The doctors would not let me in at first, but finally I carried out the work and we took the doll to the cemetery where it was buried in a grave. Instead of burying the child we buried the doll. The child was taken home a few days later and has been healthy until today.

After converting to the Pentecostal Church, Teresa got another view of the life switch: "It was a good thing that we saved the child's life, but if you step on something that has been used for a cambio de vida, you can become ill or die. Someone who is not supposed to become sick will receive the illness and die. It's really something bad. A cambio de vida also causes anxiety at the hospital, and people become afraid because they know what a cambio de vida is; that it can be done with another person in the next bed who may die."

Five years ago, Teresa had an "experience with God," she says. One day at her workplace, where she is a cleaning woman, she had a vision of a white man dressed in a white robe who told her to accept the Word of God and read the Bible. Two years earlier, her daughter and son-in-law had given up their santería practice and joined the Pentecostal Church: "My daughter and her husband also wanted me to convert. First, I didn't want to listen, and I told them to leave my house. We were fighting and arguing. Then, after my vision, I also converted."

She brought all her santería, palo monte, and espiritismo objects to the forest and left them there. Today, Teresa talks about santería and palo monte

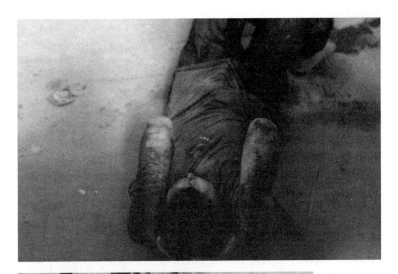

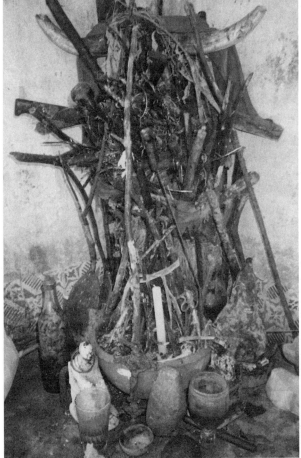

Above: Fig. 16. A man crawling on his back to the Church of San Lazaro. Photo by Johan Wedel.

Left: Fig. 17. The prenda or nganga used in palo monte. The prenda, which is said to be alive, carries out the wishes of its owner. Photo by Johan Wedel.

as the work of the Christian devil. When she gave up her old faith she became ill for one month, and, according to her, it was Satan that took advantage of the fact that she was weak. Her asthma became much worse and she got more pain in her leg than she had had before.

> I went to the church where the [Pentecostal] priest began to pray for me. He put his hand on my forehead, and I felt that something inside me went away and I fell to the floor. After that my health became much better. I have never had an asthma attack since, and I have had my leg operated on and feel fine. After this experience I live a happy, pleasant life. I get up in the morning and thank God for the life he has given me. God does much greater and more wonderful things with us than Satan did. There are people who have lost the use of their legs who come to our church, and they become well.

> If someone who still thinks that I am a santera comes for a consultation, I say, "Come in, I will advise you," and I open the Bible and read for them. If there is a santería ceremony here in the neighborhood, we all get together and pray. In that house, no santo will descend.

Today, Teresa is very critical of santería. Like Ivan, she claims that santería priests exploit people financially and take advantage of the situation when someone is poor and ill:

> If someone is ill, the santero may say that he must make santo fast or he will die. People will struggle very hard to find the money and run from the hospital to the countryside to find the animals needed. When the peasants understand that you are looking for animals because someone is ill and really needs them, they will charge more. The santeros, who have good contacts with the peasants, buy the animals cheap and then tell you that it was very expensive.

> When a foreigner consults a santero, he may say: "You are on a really bad road (camino), and Yemayá says that you must make santo in order to open your road." Then he says that it has to be Eleggua, which is the most expensive santo to make. The santero then keeps most of the money for himself. Many times I have been to ceremonies where animals have been sacrificed and the santero says that a goat or rooster has to be taken to the forest, but he takes it to his house and eats it instead.

Teresa claims that there is much envy between godchildren and describes the relationship between godfather and godchild as an evil chain that never ends:

Santería will first give you a good and tranquil life, but then your god-mother or godfather will tell you to perform more sacrifices. You have to do it again and again. As people are desperate and poor they want to believe in the santero. He may say that you will find work in [the tourist enclave] Varadero if you give a coconut, pigeons, and a rooster to Obatalá, and some candies to Eleggua bought in the dollar store. If the godchild doesn't want to do what the godfather says, he may do some work with the godchild and cause problems within the family or at the place of work. You may find the job, but then your godfather will start telling you every five seconds that Eleggua has to "eat."

Teresa's only daughter, Olga, was also a very active practitioner of san-tería, although she never made santo. According to Olga, her mother's house was dedicated to the practice of santería, and her mother consulted people over the phone in the United States. "My mother could see what was happening and described what people had in their houses," she says.

Even her ten-year-old son became possessed with Eleggua and advised people for their problems.

We learned santería from our ancestors, our family. In this house we did everything. We prepared powders, did cambio de vida, and went to the cemetery. It had effect and things really happened. The Bible says that demonic things really have effect, especially for people who are under the influence of the devil. I was told that I was a daughter of Oshún and could have all the men I wanted, like Oshún. I could live a liberal life, like a prostitute. I was prohibited from wearing black clothes or eating calabash. The santero tells you to go to bed with twenty men because you are free. Then you catch an illness like AIDS, which is very common these days, and you die.

When Olga finally left santería she was experiencing a deep life crisis: "I used to work as a ladies' hairdresser but the salary was so bad that I quit. Because of the economic crisis, life was really a struggle. I couldn't give my son the things I wanted. Everything went bad in my life and I was preoccu-pied with everything. I became depressed and got problems with my ner-vios. I spent all my money on flowers, candles, and other [santería] things but didn't see any change. I was looking for a reason to live. I was ready to kill myself and throw myself in the sea." During this time, Olga met her future husband, David, who had recently converted to the Pentecostal Church.

After a while Olga also left santería and joined the church. Her life began to change: "My husband persuaded me to change my life. My mother's house was a house with a lot of problems, and I was always arguing with my mother. It was dark in the house even when the light was on. My child also changed. He used to be very aggressive. Today we live a very peaceful life here and I decide over my own life." Olga is also critical of how santería is used to exploit people financially. According to her, everybody will lose in the end, even the santeros:

> The santo who possesses someone may say four truths and twenty lies, but people will only listen to the truths. Then they call this "evidence" and enter into santería. First, you have to bring two candles, tomorrow two coconuts and a goat. Then you have to make santo. I have seen people who have made santo because of health problems and then died almost at once. People spend a fortune on making santo and then they die.
>
> There are santeros who make a lot of money, but the santo will take it away one way or the other. The majority of the santeros live in very unhealthy places. They are not capable of advancing materially and buying some nice furniture because they spend the money on candles, flowers, and rituals. They do not prosper spiritually, either, and are always fighting within the family. Every day they wait for their lives to change, but they die poor and lonely. If there is really something helping them, where is it? When I meet someone who is going to make santo, I tell them all this. I speak of my own and my mother's experience and tell them who we were, and who we are now, thanks to the Word of God.

Teresa's son-in-law, David, also practiced santería a few years ago. But, as with his wife, he never became initiated before he changed and became a Pentecostalist:

> I was told that I was a child of Obatalá. I am a musician, and I played in a salsa band in some of the large hotels in Havana. I really thought I was the best musician in the world. My mother-in-law "developed me" in espiritismo, and I was told that I had a spiritual protector called Ta José. I also had to "develop el brujo" [become initiated in palo monte], and make santo. At that time I was always fighting and arguing with my wife and my mother-in-law.
>
> A friend brought me to a mass at the Pentecostal Church, and after some time I began to follow the Word of God. Now, we have all found the road of God and everything is very peaceful. We threw out five

sacks of sorcery stuff from this house—"prepared" dolls, iron caul-drons, powders, and all that. After that I felt very relieved. The peace of God has changed me. We don't blame any special santero or babalao for all the problems that santería may cause. It's the evil force behind that is bad.

In a similar case, Isabel, an Afro-Cuban woman in her early forties who lives in Matanzas, left santería for financial reasons:

I was born and raised in a religious family with many santeros. Almost everybody in my family has made santo. As a child I was very thin and always sick. When I was playing I sometimes felt a cold shivering and something similar to epileptic seizures, but it was not epilepsy. It was something unnatural. I was brought to a santero who said that I had to make santo. When I was seven years old I made Yemayá and received some of the other santos. I also received San Lazaro to improve my health. After I made santo the strange shivering and the attacks ceased.

With the help of my parents I always attended my santos and gave them their food [offerings and sacrifices]. Until five years ago I always took care of them. I spent the little money I had on my santos, but I never got anything back. I could never afford to buy shoes or clothe my two children. I just had enough money to buy food, and I felt sorry for them. We received clothes from our neighbors, who were not religious [santería followers] and who lived better lives than us.

Everything was for the santos, but they never helped me with any-thing, so I said, "To hell with these santos." I put everything in a sack and threw it in the garbage. My family cried to high heaven. All the followers and santeros began to criticize me, and they waited for the worst possible thing to happen.

When Isabel left santería, a friend persuaded her to visit the Pentecostal Church in the city. She began to attend their meetings and became a con-vert. After a short time, a hurricane hit Matanzas and left parts of the city under water. At the time, Isabel was living in a run-down neighborhood where the main river runs out into the open sea. The water rapidly rose and entered her house.

The water stood about a meter high in my house. Everything was float-ing: the bed, the chairs, the sofa, everything. I was stunned. Everybody told me that Yemayá had punished me for throwing away the santos.

But God is great, because after four or five months the state gave me a new, good apartment in another neighborhood with three bedrooms, living room, patio, bathroom, and kitchen with gas. Before, I used to cook with coal. Of all the bad things that I thought could occur, the best thing happened.

In the past five years my life has changed completely. I don't think about chickens, cockerels, goats, sheep, or ducks [for sacrifice], and I am doing fine. My children have grown up and they live the same life as everybody else. They are not rich, but they are healthy and live well. The rest of my family continues with the same backwardness [santería worship], but I don't! I live in a decent house without worries, and I don't want to hear anything about santos or santeros.

I now serve God in the church. What a difference! God does not ask for anything. In the [Pentecostal] church we are all sisters and brothers and we share the bread and assist each other. We help each other when someone is sick. It's very pure and nobody gossips about anybody. This is the house of God.

In Isabel's story, the santos never let her prosper economically despite her efforts, sacrifices, and worship. Ivan, Teresa, Olga, and David tell of similar experiences but go one step further and criticize santería for being exploitative, manipulative, and outright evil. In these narratives, all the perceived advantages of santería worship and practice are turned upside down, and the dark side of santería is exposed.

In their versions, people who are ill and desperately looking for a cure are made to suffer more instead of being healed. Instead of offering mutual aid between a godfather and his godchild, and a new "family" for the devotee, initiation results in a situation of dominance and dependence, which, in turn, leads to unscrupulous, financial exploitation. Instead of bringing peace, santería causes tension and stress. Instead of giving a sense of security, it causes a fear of life switches in hospitals (which may also result in people waiting to seek medical care until they are very ill or leaving the hospital too early). Santería is also said to cause anxiety and fear of stepping on objects in the streets that a santero has performed a work with.

In conclusion, both in the narratives by people who have left santería and among active santeros, one can find a similar critique: santería is often used to exploit people. The santeros relate this to the difficult economic situation while the Pentecostalists see it as part of the nature of santería. Interestingly, neither Ivan nor Teresa and her family deny that santería rituals have effect, although they argue that the social relations acquired through santería lead to exploitation of people who are often poor, desperate, and ill.

The critique presented here comes mainly from people who are, or have been, practicing santería and from followers of some of the free churches, like Jehovah's Witnesses or the Pentecostal Church. Santería is no longer perceived to be a threat to the government, and few would argue that santería is a thing of the past, or accuse it of being unscientific, irrational, or against Marxist ideas. Afro-Cuban religions and folklore have instead become good commodities for the tourist industry.

The claim that santería is unscientific and irrational is a form of misdirected critique. The santería logic may not follow Western scientific, biomedical reasoning, but its practice is based on empirical observations. The rituals performed in order to heal and avoid illnesses and other problems make good sense in terms of santería beliefs about etiology. Santería priests have good reasons for what they do, and they achieve desired effects and results in terms of healing (see ch. 5). Frequently, santería healing also results in curing, that is, in the elimination of a disease or disorder.

The critique that reduces santería practices to a form of economic activity must also be viewed in the proper context. Santería priests often compete for clients and may have good reasons for claiming that other priests cannot be trusted or that they exploit people, but they do not, of course, criticize santería per se. For those who practice Pentecostalism it is different: santería is by nature evil and bad. To think otherwise would be to go against the beliefs of their church. The critics who belong to free churches are nevertheless hugely outnumbered by the santería followers.

The economic aspects of santería have become more important with the economic crisis. It is therefore not surprising that the critique focuses mainly on economic issues. As society at large has become more commercialized and competitive, and a growing number of foreigners spend money on rituals and all kinds of work, there are more people who try to make a profit out of santería. Among those who know little about santería, and among some Marxists and academics, there are similar critical voices. Most people who are not involved in santería, however, are either just skeptical or neutral and do not exclude the possibility of turning to santería to resolve a serious problem.

Despite the critique and the fact that santería has become a rather expensive religion, it is a mass phenomenon, particularly common in poor working-class neighborhoods where many Afro-Cubans reside. Santería has become a source of spiritual power and protection. It offers health, a direction in life, relief from suffering, and a way to counter uncertainty caused by the economic crisis. For many, entry into santería also means following an ancient tradition and the beliefs of the ancestors, while at the same time acquiring a new view of how the world is constituted.

8

Conclusion

From the time of slavery until the present economic crisis in Cuba, the religious tradition that has become known as santería has meant health, protection, and a meaningful life for many Cubans. The formation of Santería, its survival and success, is related to its vast healing knowledge, adaptability to different conditions, and capacity to borrow from, and absorb, different traditions. Today in Cuba, many turn to santería because of illnesses and problems related to social and economic insecurity, problems that have grown with the economic crisis that began in 1990.

Initiates today can be found over the whole spectrum of society, and their backgrounds and professions vary. Santería exists in both poor and more wealthy neighborhoods. As indicated by the narratives, though, devotees are often Afro-Cubans from a working-class background. The religion is more common in low-income neighborhoods dominated by Afro-Cubans. It is strongest in the western provinces of Matanzas and Havana, the part of Cuba where the religion originated and where most Yoruba slaves settled.

At the beginning of the twentieth century, santería was considered to be sorcery and therefore evil. During the first two decades after the 1959 revolution, santería practice was labeled irrational and unscientific. Practitioners were controlled, and santería was discouraged because of its informal economical activities that escaped state control. In the late 1970s, the government began to present Afro-Cuban religions as folklore instead of religion. Followers were still persecuted, and santería's tolerance of alternative lifestyles was criticized. Santería was associated with backwardness in contrast to the new, modern, revolutionary Cuba.

In the mid-1980s, the situation began to change as Cuba gradually opened up toward the outside world. Private markets were permitted, investment by foreign companies was encouraged, and a tourist industry was established. In this new era, religious practice in general became better tolerated, particularly when a book about the religious life of Fidel Castro was published. During this time, the spiritual leader of the Nigerian Yoruba visited Cuba, and some babalao priests became organized for the first time into an institutionalized group.

The government further relaxed its attitude toward religious believers during the 1990s. Cuba was no longer an atheist state, and religious believers were admitted as members of the Communist Party. Exchanges and communication with the Yoruba in West Africa continued. When the Fourth International Congress of Orisha Tradition and Culture took place in Havana in 1992, delegates from Nigeria and Benin were among the invited.

The Cuban government has today adopted a more tolerant stance toward Afro-Cuban religions. Santería is flourishing, and both Cubans and foreigners spend large amounts of money on rituals and initiations, often in order to become healed from an illness. Some may themselves later initiate others. Afro-Cuban dance, music, and other artistic expressions have become important in the Cuban tourist industry and attract tourists from all over the Americas and from Europe. This interest in Afro-Cuban religion and folklore brings hard currency to Cuba and is probably an important reason behind the government's relaxed attitude toward santería.

The Roman Catholic Church in Cuba has traditionally looked upon santería with skepticism, considering it to be an obscure religious practice. This is still the officially held view, but as many santería followers consider themselves Catholic and visit churches, some priests today invite devotees and turn a blind eye to santería activities in the church.

A less tolerant attitude from the church authorities toward santería was evident when Pope John Paul II visited Cuba in 1988. The pope met with representatives of the Catholic, Protestant, and Jewish faiths. A group of babalao priests, though, was not allowed to meet the pope. Many santería followers were greatly disappointed and felt marginalized by the whole ecumenical community.

In general, few Catholics today criticize santería. Instead, its main critics are often santería practitioners themselves and people who belong to some of the free churches. They argue that santería is frequently used to exploit people financially, and they contend that some priests are more interested in earning money than in helping people. Naturally, the santería priests do not criticize santería per se as do followers of, for example, the Pentecostal churches. Many practitioners agree that santería has become more commercialized, but few would reduce its practice to a form of economic activity used to exploit people. For most people, santería addresses deeply meaningful and existential questions about suffering, illness, and social relations.

Healing can be examined from many different perspectives. I have tried to make sense of santería religious healing in relation to history, social change, cosmology, and biomedicine ("Western medicine") and, most importantly, in relation to people's own experiences. The study adopts a phenomenological perspective emphasizing embodied experience and narratives—people telling their stories in their own words. Following this approach, I have focused on particular persons in particular situations, their own interpretations of their practices, and what their beliefs have accomplished for them, not only in relation to illness and healing, but also to a larger whole, to other events in life. By focusing on how santería healing feels from the inside, from a personal and "emic" point of view, and by emphasizing the deeply religious and meaningful dimensions of people's experiences of healing, I have aimed at an understanding of how the world is "remade" for someone who turns to santería in the case of illness. I believe this approach to be fruitful for an understanding of how santería healing works.

As with the Yoruba-derived Afro-Brazilian religion candomblé (Sjørslev 2001:141), santería implies becoming "part of something bigger" where the divinities are both part of a tradition and a source of creative thinking. Santería offers a sense of wholeness because it relates illness and healing to the subjective otherworld of divinities and spirits, and to the social world of the sufferer. Instead of downplaying the social origin of sickness and viewing it as a disturbed biological process, as is common in biomedicine, the reshaping of social relations in santería is part of the healing process. It is recognized that the social environment often plays a critical role both in defining and healing sickness. Harmony must be restored in life if health is to be achieved.

Healing in santería means to recognize the importance of social relations, both in terms of new forms of social support and in terms of social explanations (such as when illness is understood as originating in disturbed relations and sorcery). Santería healing also implies taking advantage of the healing properties of many herbs and plants. However, most importantly, santería healing means to develop a relation to the santería world, a world manifested in a rich mythology, complex divination systems, elaborated rituals, and nature itself.

To become involved in santería because of a health problem, or for any other reason, is to begin to approach the otherworld of divinities and spirits. Santería healing is a process in which a person begins to understand illness from a different perspective and establishes and takes part in an exchange with the world of the santería divinities. In this new perception of the world, the divinities are "given" offerings, sacrifices, and drum ceremonies, and in return "give back" health and prosperity. The gradual process of healing in santería is based on relations and encounters with the divine world where the divine force (ashé) is present in plants and sacred stones, music and prayers, and sacrificial blood and in the bodies of humans during possession trance.

The relationship with the divinities is especially important when someone goes through initiation because the initiate will form a close relation and "give his head" to a specific santo. This divinity will, in turn, protect and heal the initiate. The initiation ritual is often performed when someone is suffering from a serious illness, but initiation is more than a way of treating illness. It is a process through which a person will experience a transformation of the self. Santería will reshape the world for the initiate, who, in turn, will experience the world in a new, sacred, and deeply meaningful way.

Through this transformation, the initiate will relate to nature in a different, more intense way, because nature is given a new meaning. He will also relate to other humans in novel ways and develop a new understanding of what has provoked his illness and what may cause problems and illness in the future. The initiation becomes a deeply meaningful and enriching ontological journey, an existential voyage in which the whole being is affected. In the process, the initiate not only acquires new social relations but may also begin to view sickness as deriving from the social environment and strained social relations.

Santería offers both a different etiology and different treatment of sickness. Healing is grounded in bodily experience, and when healing takes place through initiation, the ill person has to be active and not only perform the prescribed rituals but also follow pragmatic and "this-worldly" directives given by the divinities in order to become well. The outcome of the healing process is not definitive, is often achieved gradually, and is dependent on the subjective experience of the person being healed; a person may feel healed even if the underlying biological or biochemical problem remains the same. By understanding mind, body, and social relations as interwoven with one another, and by recognizing the role of healing as grounded in a bodily experience, the whole person becomes part of the healing process.

Santería healing is based on the assumption that illness can be provoked, avoided, and expelled by supernatural agents. In this view, there are no clear boundaries between mind and body, self and others. Illness is not seen as something that takes place in isolation, and illness occurs not only in the body. Illness and healing are part of, and dependent on, the ill person's current situation, personal history, social environment, the divinity who "owns" the person's head, the personal sign or letra, and, in general, relations to other humans, divinities, and spirits. Each illness is unique in the same way as each healing procedure is unique and dependent on the context. To recognize that each illness is unique is also to recognize that each person's way to health, prosperity, and happiness is unique.

Through santería healing, illness is turned into a constructive and positive experience; the individual is not only given the possibility to begin a new life, but he or she will also get access to new forms of knowledge and divine power that may be used to heal others. Illness, then, is also potentially a source of healing knowledge, knowledge that is only accessible to the devotees.

The santería view of illness is especially important when people suffer from illnesses that are biomedically unspecified, such as nervous problems, but it is significant in all cases of illness, physical as well as psychological in origin. The reasons why Cubans and people from all over the world turn to santería in order to become healed from illness must be understood in relation to a fundamental fact: santería transforms the experience of illness and gives meaning to illness and suffering in ways that biomedicine cannot. According to santería ideas, biomedicine addresses one, albeit important, aspect of suffering when locating illness in the physical body or the mind. However, in order to achieve well-being, santería adopts a more holistic perspective, acknowledging also sacred and spiritual dimensions of illness.

Santería is today becoming prevalent not only in Cuba but all over the New World. The religion is gathering many followers even in Europe. Other Yoruba-derived traditions, such as candomblé, are also popular, especially in the Brazilian state of Bahia. In southwestern Nigeria, the Yoruba religion still constitutes an important part of many people's lives. In all those places, the healing of illness forms an important part of religious practice.

Santería healing touches upon a whole series of universally compelling and challenging ideas about well-being and recovery from illness: healing through a gradual transformation of the self; the creation of a relationship between humans and a spirit-world; the interpenetration of mind and body, individuality, and social relations; activity rather than passivity; and the view of healing as more of a process than a specific event. Some of these ideas and practices can also be found in other healing traditions and are significant when developing more general notions about healing. As in the West, more and more people are turning to various forms of non-Western healing and "alternative medicine." Knowledge of such traditions represents not only a challenge to Western medical theory but also an important contribution to an understanding of the human condition.

Appendix 1. Herbs and Plants

Vernacular name	English name	Scientific name
Abrecamino	Siguaraya	*Trichilia havanensia. Jacq.*
Álamo	Poplar	*Ficus religiosa. L.*
Albahaca	Basil	*Ocimum basilicum. L.*
Algodón	Cotton plant	*Gossypium barbadense. L.*
Almácigo	Gum tree	*Bursera simaruba. Sarg.*
Almendra	Indian almond	*Terminalia catappa. L.*
Berro	Watercress	*Nasturtium officinale. R. Br.*
Canutillo	Day flower	*Commelina elegans. H.B.K.*
Ceiba	Silk-cotton tree	*Ceiba pentandra. L.*
Escoba amarga	Feverfew	*Parthenium hysterophorus. L.*
Galán de día	Day-blooming jasmine	*Cestrum diurnum. L.*
Granada	Pomegranate	*Punica granatum. L.*
Guásima	Bastard cedar	*Guazuma tomentosa. H.B.K.*
Jía brava	—	*Casearia aculeata. Jacq.*
Mastuerzo	Common cress	*Lipidiun virginicum. L.*
Muralla	Orange jasmine	*Murraya paniculata. L.*
Paraíso	Chinaberry tree	*Melia azederach. L.*
Pata de Gallina	Star shake	*Eleusine indica. L. Gaerth.*
Pimienta	Pepper	*Piper nigrum. L.*
Piñón de botija	Purging nut	*Jatropha curcas. L.*
Platanillo de cuba	Spiked pepper	*Piper aduncum. L.*
Quimbombó	Okra	*Hibicus esculentus. L.*
Rascabarriga	—	*Espadaea amoena. A. Rich.*
Romerillo	Beggar's ticks	*Bidens pilosa. L.*
Rompezaragüey	Siam weed	*Eupatorium odoratum. L.*
Ruda	Herb of grace	*Ruta chalepensis. L.*
Sábila	Aloes	*Aloe vera. L.*

Vernacular name	English name	Scientific name
Salvadera	Sandbox tree	*Hura crepitana. L.*
Salvia	Sage	*Pluchea adorata. Cass.*
Sasafrás	Sassafras	*Bursera graveolens. Triana y Planch.*
Vencedor	—	*Zanthoxylum pistacifolium. Griseb.*
Yerba mora	Nightshade	*Solanum nigrum. L.*
Zapote	Sapota tree	*Sapota Achras. Mill.*

Appendix 2. An Examination of Santería Consultations

A sample of one hundred santería consultations were examined. The consultations had been with a santería priest who performed using the dilogún divination system with cowrie shells. The study focused on the reason for the consultation, the supposed cause of the problem, recommendations by the santero, and gender distribution. Results:

1. What was the reason for the consultation (according to the priest)?

Illness	54
Family problems	23
Problems with the law	14
Other reasons	9

2. What caused the client's problem?

Sorcery	42
"Punishment" by a santo	3
Other	55

3. What did the santero recommend (one or more of the following)?

Spiritual cleansing or bath	96
Visit to a biomedical doctor	68
Ritual to receive necklace/warriors	67
Offering or sacrifice	55
Become initiated (make santo)	42

4. Of the 54 who visited the santero because of illness, one or more of the following was recommended:

Spiritual cleansing or bath	54	(100%)
Visit to a biomedical doctor	51	(94%)
Offering or sacrifice	40	(74%)
Ritual to receive necklace/warriors	38	(70%)
Become initiated (make santo)	25	(46%)

5. Gender distribution among clients (total):

Women	51
Men	49

6. In 54 cases, the problem was illness. Gender distribution:

Women	28	(52%)
Men	26	(48%)

7. Gender distribution among those with family problems:

Women	13	(57%)
Men	10	(43%)

8. Gender distribution among those with legal problems:

Women	3	(21%)
Men	11	(79%)

9. In 42 cases, the problem was related to sorcery. Gender distribution:

Women	20	(48%)
Men	22	(52%)

10. In 42 cases, the client was advised to become initiated (make santo). Gender distribution:

Women	24	(57%)
Men	18	(43%)

Appendix 3. List of Narrators

Name (pseudonym)	Age	Descent	Place of residence	Occupation	Type of practitioner
A.M.	Late 30s	Hispanic	Havana	Physician, Ifá priest	Babalao
Amelia (Eva's daughter)	10	Hispanic	Matanzas	Student	None
Ana	Mid 40s	Afro-Cuban	Havana	Cashier	Santera, spiritist
Antonio (Eva's husband)	Late 40s	Hispanic	Matanzas	Engineer	None
David (Olga's husband)	Early 30s	Hispanic	Havana	Musician	Pentecostal church practitioner (formerly spiritist)
Diana	Mid 30s	Hispanic	Matanzas	Receptionist	None
Elena	Mid 20s	Afro-Cuban	Havana	Unemployed	Santera
Eva	Mid 40s	Hispanic	Matanzas	Unemployed	Santera, spiritist
Florencia (Matilda's daughter)	Mid 20s	Afro-Cuban	Matanzas	Cleaner	None
Ivan	Mid 40s	Hispanic	Havana	Unemployed	Pentecostal church practitioner (formerly santero, palero)
Isabel	Early 40s	Afro-Cuban	Matanzas	Unemployed	Pentecostal church practitioner (formerly santera)
Julio	Mid 50s	Afro-Cuban	Havana	Ifá priest	Babalao
Lidia	Mid 30s	Afro-Cuban	Havana	Housewife	Santera

(continued)

Appendix 3—*Continued*

Name (pseudonym)	Age	Descent	Place of residence	Occupation	Type of practitioner
Lucia	Mid 30s	Afro-Cuban	Matanzas	Secretary	Santera
Luis	Mid 50s	Hispanic	Havana	Retired, Ifá priest	Babalao
María	Mid 40s	Hispanic	Matanzas	Storekeeper	Jehovah's Witness practitioner (formerly santería devotee)
Mario (Silvia's husband)	Early 30s	Hispanic	Havana	Baker	Santero
Matilda (Oscar's wife)	Early 50s	Afro-Cuban	Matanzas	Storekeeper	Santera
Máximo (Eva's godfather)	Early 50s	Afro-Cuban	Matanzas	Santería priest	Santero, palero, spiritist
Mercedes	Late 50s	Afro-Cuban	Havana	Retired	Santera
Olga (Teresa's daughter)	Early 30s	Afro-Cuban	Havana	Unemployed	Pentecostal church practitioner (formerly santera, spiritist)
Oscar (Matilda's husband)	Early 50s	Afro-Cuban	Matanzas	Unemployed	Santero, spiritist
Patricia (Julio's godchild)	Mid 50s	Afro-Cuban	Havana	Retired	Santería devotee (not initiated)
Reina	Late 20s	Afro-Cuban	Germany/ Havana	Student	Santería devotee (not initiated)
Rosa (Julio's godchild)	Mid 20s	Afro-Cuban	Havana	Receptionist	Spiritist, santería devotee (not initiated)
Silvia (Mario's wife)	Early 30s	Afro-Cuban	Havana	Unemployed	Santera
Teresa (Olga's mother)	Early 50s	Afro-Cuban	Havana	Cleaner	Pentecostal church practitioner (formerly santera, palera, spiritist)

Notes

Introduction

1. Unless otherwise noted, all translations from Spanish are my own.

Chapter 1. The Struggle against Illness

1. I will use the term "sorcery" when discussing magical "works" and distinguish it from "witchcraft," which often takes place on a subconscious level (cf. Kapferer 1997:8).

Chapter 2. Cuba and the Formation of Santería

1. See Thomas (1997) and Scott (1985) for a history of Cuba and the slave trade.

2. The encounters between Africans and Europeans should not be interpreted as encounters between two "bodies" of beliefs and values. The slaves cannot be said to have shared a culture in the way that the European colonists in a particular colony did. "The Africans in any New World colony in fact became a *community* and began to share a *culture* only insofar as, and as fast as, they themselves created them" (Mintz and Price 1992:14).

3. Other tribal groups brought to Cuba were the Mandinga, Arará, Gangá, Carabalí, and Congo. The Carabalí originated from west Cameroon and Calabar (southeast Nigeria). Slaves from this area established the all-male secret society Abakuá that today has many members in the cities of Matanzas, Cárdenas, and Havana. Arará is a religious tradition that can be traced back to the Ewe-Fon people of present-day Benin (Martínez Furé 1979; Ortiz 1975). Although it has its own pantheon of divinities, rituals, and drum style, it is becoming absorbed by the more widespread practice of santería. It is common that Arará priests use the santería names of the divinities. Arará priests also participate in santería rituals and vice versa.

Chapter 3. Etiology and Healing

1. Two other variants of espiritismo also exist in Cuba. These are *espiritismo de cordón*, where the participants form a circle and evoke possession trance by using body movements and singing; and *espiritismo cruzao*, where herbs and different objects are used in healing and where the participants may also be advised to carry out animal sacrifices. This practice has borrowed ideas from palo monte and is practiced mainly in and around Santiago de Cuba. Espiritismo cruzao is very far from the spiritual movement Kardecism, from which espiritismo originally developed.

2. A santero gave the following reason for this practice: "The sticks are put like a castle, like when the king walks under the arms and lances." The ceremony is only performed with the divinities who are considered to be males, such as Eleggua, Ogún, Ochosi, Shangó, and Aggayú.

Chapter 4. Pantheon and Rituals

1. See Barnes (1997) for a history of Ogún in Africa and the New World.

Chapter 5. Healing, Curing, and the Self

1. Cabrera (1993b) describes how, almost fifty years ago, sacrifices were performed in sacred lagoons. None of my informants had any knowledge of this practice being carried out today.

2. Interestingly, the words "holy," "whole," and "health" share the same etymology (Rappaport 1979:234).

Glossary

Aggayú: A santería divinity. Lord of the volcanoes and the barren plain.

Aguán: Spiritual cleansing ritual related to the divinity San Lazaro (Babalú Ayé).

Ahijado, Ahijada: Godchild of a santería priest.

Aña: Spirit that resides in the largest of the three sacred batá drums.

Aro or **Ano**: Sickness.

Ashé: Divine power and force of life; luck; prosperity; a powder used during initiation.

Asiento: Literally "seating," when a santería divinity is "put in the head" of the devotee.

Babalao: High priest of santería.

Babalocha: Male santero who has initiated others.

Babalú Ayé: A santería divinity and lord of skin ailments, infectious diseases, and illness in general. He is commonly known as San Lazaro.

Baño de desenvolvimiento: Bath for spiritual development.

Batá: Sacred drums.

Bembé: Drum feast for the santería divinities.

Bóveda: Spiritist table.

Brujería: Sorcery; the palo monte religion; all kinds of magic activities.

Cabildos: Societies for free slaves during the nineteenth century.

Cambio de vida: "Life switch." Magic in which the "life force" of two persons is switched.

Canastillero: Shelved cabinet where the santería religious objects are placed.

Casa-templo: The home of a santería priest where religious objects are also kept and where rituals take place.

Cascarilla: Pulverized eggshells used in many santería rituals.

Cofá de Orula: Ritual related to the lord of divination, Orula, performed for females.

Collar: Beaded necklace with colors that correspond to a certain santería divinity.

Comida para la tierra: "Food to the earth." A ritual performed in order to avoid death.

Cuarto de santo: Prepared room for the santería initiation.

Despojo: Ritual cleansing.

Dilogún: Divination system with cowrie shells.

Ebbó: Offering or sacrifice.

Eleggua: A santería divinity and lord of crossroads. He opens and closes the ways of life for humans.

Ekpuelé: Divination chain used by the babalao, high priest of santería.

Espiritismo: Spiritism. Religious tradition that focuses on communication with spirits.

Espiritismo de mesa: Common variant of spiritism in which the participants sing and pray in front of a table with spiritist objects.

Espiritista: Practitioner of spiritism.

Ewe: Herbs and plants.

Garabato: Hooked staff, the symbol of Eleggua.

Hacer santo: To "make saint," to become initiated into santería.

Ibeyis: Divine twins of the santería pantheon.

Ibo: Divination objects.

Ifá: Divination system of the babalao, high priest of santería.

Igbodu: Prepared room for the santería initiation.

Ikú: Death.

Ilé: Santería household.

Inle: A santería divinity related to fishing and hunting.

Iré: Positive or good.

Itá: Divination.

Italero: Divination expert.

Itótele: Middle one of the three sacred batá drums.

Ituto: Funeral ceremony.

Iyá: Largest of the three sacred batá drums.

Iyabó: Santería initiate who must obey certain rules for a period of one year.

Iyalocha: Female santera who has initiated others.

Letra or Odu: Outcome of the divination process.

Limpieza: Ritual cleansing.

Lucumí: People of Yoruba descent; santería ritual language; santería.

Madrina: Godmother.

Mal de ojo: Evil eye.

Mano de Orula: Ritual related to the lord of divination, Orula, performed for males.

Medio asiento: Santería halfway initiation that is often carried out in cases of severe illness.

Misa espiritual: Spiritual mass.

Moyubbar: To pray in the santería ritual language Lucumí.

Muerto: Spirit of the dead.

Muerto oscuro: Spirit that lacks light and may do harm.

Nervios: Literally "nerves," a folk syndrome of emotional stress.

Obatalá: A santería divinity and the lord of peace, purity, and justice.

Obba: A santería divinity and wife of Shangó.

Obí: Coconut. Divination instrument and mythological being.

Ochosi: A santería divinity and the lord of hunting.

Oddudua or **Oddua**: A santería divinity related to purity.

Ogún: A santería divinity and the lord of iron.

Okónkolo: Smallest of the three sacred batá drums.

Olodumare: Supreme god and creator.

Olofi: Aspect of Olodumare.

Olokun: A Santería divinity who represents the ocean depths, often evoked in order to heal illness.

Omiero: Juice of sacred herbs.

Oriaté: Song leader during santería rituals.

Orisha: Santería divinity or santo.

Orishaoko: A santería divinity and the lord of agriculture.

Oru: Ritual order.

Orula or **Orunmila**: A santería divinity and the lord of divination.

Osain: A santería divinity and the lord of plants and herbs.

Osainista: Expert on plants and herbs and their properties.

Oshún: A santería divinity related to rivers, freshwater, and love.

Osobo: Negative or bad.

Ósun: A santería divinity that protects the devotee.

Otán: Sacred stone that represents a particular santería divinity.

Oyá: A santería divinity related to the cemetery; and queen of the wind.

Padrino: Godfather.

Palenque: Community for runaway slaves during colonial rule in Cuba.

Palero, **Palera**: Palo monte priest, priestess.

Palo monte: Religious tradition with roots in the Congo.

Pañuelo: A cloth used to cover the soup tureens where the santería objects are kept.

Patakies: Myths about divinities and spirits related to the divination systems.

Pinaldo: Ritual where the right to sacrifice large animals is obtained.

Prenda or **nganga**: Iron cauldron used in palo monte.

Prenda cristiana: Iron cauldron used for well-being in palo monte.

Prenda judía: Iron cauldron used for evil work in palo monte.

Regla de Ocha: Santería.

Resguardo: Protective talisman.

Rogación de cabeza: Ritual performed in order to acquire balance and harmony.

Rompimiento: Literally "breakage." Ritual act carried out in order to take away an evil, disturbing spirit.

San Lazaro: A santería divinity and lord of skin ailments, infectious diseases, and illness in general. Also known as Babalú Ayé.

Santero, Santera: Santería priest, priestess.

Santo: Orisha or santería divinity.

Shangó: A santería divinity related to thunder, lightning, and manly beauty.

Sopera: Soup tureen containing the sacred stones, otánes.

Tambor: Drum ceremony.

Trabajo: Spiritual work.

Warriors: The santería divinities Ogún, Ochosi, and Ósun, who are said to walk together with Eleggua.

Yemayá: A santería divinity and queen of the oceans.

Yerbero: Herbalist; store with herbs and santería and palo monte objects.

Yewa: A santería divinity related to virginity and to the cemetery.

Bibliography

Amarasingham Rhodes, Lorna. 1996. Studying Biomedicine as a Cultural System. In *Medical Anthropology: Contemporary Theory and Method,* edited by Carolyn F. Sargent and Thomas M. Johnson. Rev. ed. Westport, Conn.: Praeger.

American Association for World Health. 1998. Denial of Food and Medicine: The Impact of the U.S. Embargo on Health and Nutrition in Cuba. An executive summary, edited by Julia Sweig and Kai Bird. In *Health and Nutrition in Cuba: Effects of the U.S. Embargo.* Stockholm: Olof Palme International Center.

Argüelles Mederos, Anibal, and Ileana Hodge Limonta. 1991. *Los llamados cultos sincréticos y el espiritismo: Estudio monográfico sobre su significación social en la sociedad cubana contemporánea.* Havana: Editorial Academia.

Ayensu, Edward S. 1981. *Medicinal Plants of the West Indies.* Algonac, Mich.: Reference Publications.

Barnes, Sandra T., ed. 1997. *Africa's Ogun: Old World and New.* 2d, expanded ed. Bloomington: Indiana University Press.

Barnet, Miguel. 1983. *La fuente viva.* Havana: Editorial Letras Cubanas.

———. 1988. Algunas palabras necesarias. *Arieto* 1:5–7.

Bascom, William R. 1952. Two Forms of Afro-Cuban Divination. In *Acculturation in the Americas,* edited by Sol Tax. Chicago: University of Chicago Press.

———. 1969. *Ifa Divination: Communication between Gods and Men in West Africa.* Bloomington: Indiana University Press.

———. 1980. *Sixteen Cowries: Yoruba Divination from Africa to the New World.* Bloomington: Indiana University Press.

Bastide, Roger. 1971. *African Civilisations in the New World.* Translated from the French by Peter Green. New York: Harper and Row.

Benkomo, Juan. 2000. Crafting the Sacred *Batá* Drums. In *Afro-Cuban Voices: On Race and Identity in Contemporary Cuba,* edited by Pedro Pérez Sarduy and Jean Stubbs. Gainesville: University Press of Florida.

Bolívar, Natalia. 1990. *Los orishas en Cuba.* Havana: Ediciones Unión.

Bourguignon, Erika. 1973. *Religion, Altered States of Consciousness, and Social Change.* Columbus: Ohio State University Press.

Brandon, George. 1990. Sacrificial Practices in Santeria, an African-Cuban Religion in the United States. In *Africanisms in American Culture*, edited by Joseph E. Holloway. Bloomington: Indiana University Press.

———. 1991. The Uses of Plants in Healing in an Afro-Cuban Religion, Santeria. *Journal of Black Studies* 22(1):55–76.

———. 1993. *Santeria from Africa to the New World: The Dead Sell Memories.* Bloomington: Indiana University Press.

———. 2002. Hierarchy without a Head: Observations on Changes in the Social Organization of Some Afroamerican Religions in the United States, 1959–1999, with Special Reference to Santeria. *Archives de Sciences sociales des Religions* 117:151–74.

Brown, David H. 1996. Toward an Ethnoaesthetics of Santería Ritual Arts: The Practice of Altar-Making and Gift Exchange. In *Santería Aesthetics in Contemporary Latin American Art*, edited by Arturo Lindsay. Washington, D.C.: Smithsonian Institution Press.

Buckley, Anthony D. 1985. *Yoruba Medicine.* Oxford: Clarendon Press.

Butterworth, Douglas. 1974. Grass-Roots Political Organization in Cuba: A Case of the Committees for the Defense of the Revolution. In *Latin American Urban Research: Anthropological Perspectives on Latin American Urbanization*, edited by Wayne A. Cornelius and Felicity M. Trueblood. Beverly Hills, Calif.: Sage.

———. 1980. *People of Buena Ventura: Relocation of Slum Dwellers in Post-revolutionary Cuba.* Urbana: University of Illinois Press.

Cabrera, Lydia. 1993a [1954]. *El monte.* Havana: Editorial Letras Cubanas.

———. 1993b [1973]. *La laguna sagrada de San Joaquín.* Miami: Ediciones Universal.

Canizares, Raul. 1993. *Walking with the Night: The Afro-Cuban World of Santeria.* Rochester, Vt.: Destiny Books.

———. 1994. Santeria: From Afro-Caribbean Cult to World Religion. *Caribbean Quarterly* 40(1):59–63.

Carrithers, Michael, Steven Collins, and Steven Lukes, eds. 1985. *The Category of the Person: Anthropology, Philosophy, History.* Cambridge: Cambridge University Press.

Castellanos, Isabel. 1996. From Ulkumí to Lucumí: A Historical Overview of Religious Acculturation in Cuba. In *Santería Aesthetics in Contemporary Latin American Art*, edited by Arturo Lindsay. Washington, D.C.: Smithsonian Institution Press.

Castellanos, Jorge, and Isabel Castellanos. 1988. *Cultura afrocubana 1: El negro en Cuba, 1492–1844.* Miami: Ediciones Universal.

———. 1992. *Cultura afrocubana 3: Las religiones y las lenguas.* Miami: Ediciones Universal.

———. 1994. *Cultura afrocubana 4: Letras, música, arte.* Miami: Ediciones Universal.

Castro, Fidel. 1987. *Fidel and Religion: Talks with Frei Betto.* Havana: Publications Office of the Council of State.

Cohen, Anthony P. 1994. *Self Consciousness: An Alternative Anthropology of Identity.* London: Routledge.

Csordas, Thomas J. 1987. Health and the Holy in African and Afro-American Spirit Possession. *Social Science and Medicine* 24(1):1–11.

———. 1994. *The Sacred Self: A Cultural Phenomenology of Charismatic Healing.* Berkeley: University of California Press.

———. 1996. Imaginal Performance and Memory in Ritual Healing. In *The Performance of Healing,* edited by Carol Laderman and Marina Roseman. London: Routledge.

Csordas, Thomas J., and Arthur Kleinman. 1996. The Therapeutic Process. In *Medical Anthropology: Contemporary Theory and Method,* edited by Carolyn F. Sargent and Thomas M. Johnson. Rev. ed. Westport, Conn.: Praeger.

Curry, Mary C. 1997. *Making the Gods in New York: The Yoruba Religion in the African American Community.* New York: Garland Publishing.

Cuyás, Arturo, and Antonio Cuyás. 1960. *Gran diccionario Cuyás.* Edicion Revolucionaria. Instituto Cubano del Libro.

Daniel, Yvonne. 1995. *Rumba: Dance and Social Change in Contemporary Cuba.* Bloomington: Indiana University Press.

Desjarlais, Robert R. 1992. *Body and Emotion: The Aesthetics of Illness and Healing in the Nepal Himalayas.* Philadelphia: University of Pennsylvania Press.

Dianteill, Erwan. 2000. *Des dieux et des signes: Initiation, écriture et divination dans les religions afro-cubaines.* Paris: Éditions de l'École des hautes études en sciences sociales.

Díaz Fabelo, Teodoro. 1960. *Olorun.* Havana: Ediciones del Departamento de Folklore del Teatro Nacional de Cuba.

Drewal, Margaret T. 1992. *Yoruba Ritual: Performers, Play, Agency.* Bloomington: Indiana University Press.

Eckstein, Susan E. 1994. *Back From the Future: Cuba under Castro.* Princeton, N.J.: Princeton University Press.

Etkin, Nina L. 1988. Cultural Constructions of Efficacy. In *The Context of Medicines in Developing Countries: Studies in Pharmaceutical Anthropology,* edited by Sjaak van der Geest and Susan R. Whyte. Dordrecht: Kluwer.

———. 1996. Ethnopharmacology: The Conjunction of Medical Ethnography and the Biology of Therapeutic Action. In *Medical Anthropology: Contemporary Theory and Method,* edited by Carolyn F. Sargent and Thomas M. Johnson. Rev. ed. Westport, Conn.: Praeger.

Evans-Pritchard, Edward E. 1937. *Witchcraft, Oracles, and Magic among the Azande.* Oxford: Clarendon Press.

Feinsilver, Julie M. 1993. *Healing the Masses: Cuban Health Politics at Home and Abroad.* Berkeley: University of California Press.

Finkler, Kaja. 1985. *Spiritualist Healers in Mexico: Successes and Failures of Alternative Therapeutics*. South Hadley, Mass.: Praeger, Bergin and Garvey Publishers.

———. 1994. Sacred Healing and Biomedicine Compared. *Medical Anthropology Quarterly* 8(2):178–97.

Flores-Peña, Ysamur, and Roberta J. Evanchuk. 1994. *Santería Garments and Altars: Speaking without a Voice*. Jackson: University Press of Mississippi.

Friedson, Steven M. 1996. *Dancing Prophets: Musical Experience in Tumbuka Healing*. Chicago: University of Chicago Press.

Garcia Cortéz, Julio. 1983. *El Santo (la Ocha): Secretos de la religion Lucumi*. Miami: .Ediciones Universal.

Geschiere, Peter. 1997. *The Modernity of Witchcraft: Politics and the Occult in Postcolonial Africa*. Charlottesville: University Press of Virginia.

Good, Byron J. 1994. *Medicine, Rationality, and Experience: An Anthropological Perspective*. Cambridge: Cambridge University Press.

Goodman, Felicitas D. 1988. *Ecstasy, Ritual, and Alternate Reality: Religion in a Pluralistic World*. Bloomington: Indiana University Press.

———. 1990. *Where the Spirits Ride the Wind: Trance Journeys and Other Ecstatic Experiences*. Bloomington: Indiana University Press.

Granma International. 1988. Fourth Congress of Orisha Tradition and Culture Scheduled to Take Place in Havana. February 28.

Gregory, Steven. 1987. Santeria in New York City: A Study in Cultural Resistance. Ph.D. diss. Ann Arbor, Mich.: University Microfilms International.

Guanche, Jesus. 1983. *Procesos etnoculturales de Cuba*. Havana: Editorial Letras Cubanas.

Guillermoprieto, Alma. 1998. A Visit to Havana. *New York Review of Books* 45(5): 19–24.

Hagedorn, Katherine J. 2001. *Divine Utterances: The Performance of Afro-Cuban Santería*. Washington, D.C.: Smithsonian Institution Press.

Hahn, Robert A. 1995. *Sickness and Healing: An Anthropological Perspective*. New Haven, Conn.: Yale University Press.

Howard, Phillip A. 1998. *Changing History: Afro-Cuban Cabildos and Societies of Color in the Nineteenth Century*. Baton Rouge: Louisiana State University Press.

Jackson, Michael D. 1989. *Paths toward a Clearing: Radical Empiricism and Ethnographic Inquiry*. Bloomington: Indiana University Press.

———. 1996. Introduction to *Things as They Are: New Directions in Phenomenological Anthropology*, edited by Michael Jackson. Bloomington: Indiana University Press.

Jacobson-Widding, Anita. 1989. Introduction: Cultural Categories and the Power of Ambiguity. In *Culture, Experience, and Pluralism: Essays on African Ideas of Illness and Healing*, edited by Anita Jacobson-Widding and David Westerlund. Uppsala Studies in Cultural Anthropology 13. Stockholm: Almqvist and Wiksell International.

James, Edward. 1970. Introduction to *Shango de Ima: A Yoruba Mystery Play*, by Pepe

Carrul. English adaptation, with a preface by Susan Sherman and introduction by Jerome Rothenberg and Edward James. New York: Doubleday.

Jones, Michael O., Patrick A. Polk, Ysamur Flores-Peña, and Roberta J. Evanchuk. 2001. Invisible: Hospitals: Botánicas in Ethnic Health Care. In *Healing Logics: Culture and Medicine in Modern Health Belief Systems,* edited by Erika Brady. Logan: Utah State University Press.

Kapferer, Bruce. 1997. *The Feast of the Sorcerer: Practices of Consciousness and Power.* Chicago: University of Chicago Press.

Kleinman, Arthur. 1980. *Patients and Healers in the Context of Culture: An Exploration of the Borderland between Anthropology, Medicine, and Psychiatry.* Berkeley: University of California Press.

———. 1995. *Writing at the Margin: Discourse between Anthropology and Medicine.* Berkeley: University of California Press.

Lachatañeré, Rómulo. 1992. *El sistema religioso de los afrocubanos.* A compilation of previous publications. Havana: Editorial de Ciencias Sociales.

Laderman, Carol, and Marina Roseman. 1996. Introduction to *The Performance of Healing,* edited by C. Laderman and M. Roseman. London: Routledge.

Lawal, Babatunde. 1996. From Africa to the Americas: Art in Yoruba Religion. In *Santería Aesthetics in Contemporary Latin American Art,* edited by Arturo Lindsay. Washington, D.C.: Smithsonian Institution Press.

Lewis, Oscar, Ruth M. Lewis, and Susan Rigdon. 1977a. *Four Men: Living the Revolution: An Oral History of Contemporary Cuba.* Urbana: University of Illinois Press.

———. 1977b. *Four Women: Living the Revolution: An Oral History of Contemporary Cuba.* Urbana: University of Illinois Press.

———.1978. *Neighbors: Living the Revolution: An Oral History of Contemporary Cuba.* Urbana: University of Illinois Press.

Lex, Barbara. 1979. The Neurobiology of Ritual Trance. In *The Spectrum of Ritual: A Biogenetic Structural Analysis,* edited by Eugene G. d'Aquili, Charles D. Laughlin, and John McManus. New York: Columbia University Press.

Lock, Margareth, and Nancy Scheper-Hughes. 1996. A Critical-Interpretive Approach in Medical Anthropology: Rituals and Routines of Discipline and Dissent. In *Medical Anthropology: Contemporary Theory and Method,* edited by Carolyn F. Sargent and Thomas M. Johnson. Rev. ed. Westport, Conn.: Praeger.

Low, Setha M. 1994. Embodied Metaphors: Nerves as Lived Experience. In *Embodiment and Experience: The Existential Ground of Culture and Self,* edited by Thomas J. Csordas. Cambridge: Cambridge University Press.

Marks, Morton. 1987. Exploring *El Monte:* Ethnobotany and the Afro-Cuban Science of the Concrete. In *En torno a Lydia Cabrera (cincuentenario de 'cuentos negros de Cuba,' 1936–1986),* edited by Isabel Castellanos and Josefina Inclán. Miami: Ediciones Universal.

Martínez Furé, Rogelio. 1979. *Diálogos imaginarios.* Havana: Editorial Arte y Literatura.

Mason, Michael A. 1993. "The Blood That Runs through the Veins": The Creation of Identity and a Client's Experience of Cuban-American *Santería Dilogún* Divination. *The Drama Review* 37(2):119–30.

———. 1994. "I Bow My Head to the Ground": The Creation of Bodily Experience in a Cuban American *Santería* Initiation. *Journal of American Folklore* 107:23–39.

Matibag, Eugenio. 1996. *Afro-Cuban Religious Experience: Culture Reflections in Narrative.* Gainesville: University Press of Florida.

———. 1997. Ifá and Interpretation: An Afro-Caribbean Literary Practice. In *Sacred Possessions: Vodou, Santería, Obeah, and the Caribbean,* edited by Margarite Fernández Olmos and Lizabeth Paravisini-Gebert. New Brunswick, N.J.: Rutgers University Press.

Mintz, Sidney W., and Richard Price. 1992. *The Birth of African-American Culture: An Anthropological Perspective.* Boston: Beacon Press.

Montejo, Esteban. 1968. *The Autobiography of a Runaway Slave,* edited by Miguel Barnet. New York: Pantheon Books.

Moore, Carlos. 1988. *Castro, the Blacks, and Africa.* Los Angeles: University of California Center for Afro-American Studies.

Murphy, Joseph M. 1993. *Santería: African Spirits in America.* Boston: Beacon Press.

———. 1994. *Working the Spirit: Ceremonies of the African Diaspora.* Boston: Beacon Press.

Neher, Andrew. 1962. A Physiological Explanation of Unusual Behavior in Ceremonies Involving Drums. *Human Biology* 4:151–60.

Orozco, Román, and Natalia Bolívar. 1998. *Cuba Santa: Comunistas, santeros y cristianos en la isla de Fidel Castro.* Madrid: El País.

Ortiz, Fernando. 1975 [1916]. *Los negros esclavos.* Havana: Editorial de Ciencias Sociales.

———. 1992 [1921]. *Los cabildos y la fiesta afrocubanos del Día de Reyes.* Havana: Editorial de Ciencias Sociales.

———. 1995 [1906]. *Los negros brujos.* Havana: Editorial de Ciencias Sociales.

Palmié, Stephan. 1995. Against Syncretism: "Africanizing" and "Cubanizing" Discourses in North American Òrìsà Worship. In *Counterworks: Managing the Diversity of Knowledge,* edited by Richard Fardon. London: Routledge.

———. 2002. *Wizards and Scientists: Explorations in Afro-Cuban Modernity and Tradition.* Durham, N.C., and London: Duke University Press.

Pasquali, Elaine A. 1986. Santeria: A Religion That Is a Health Care System for Long Island Cuban-Americans. *Journal of the New York State Nurses Association* 17:12–15.

———. 1994. Santeria. *Journal of Holistic Nursing* 12:380–90.

Peek, Philip M. 1991. African Divination Systems: Non-Normal Modes of Cognition. In *African Divination Systems: Ways of Knowing,* edited by Philip M. Peek. Bloomington: Indiana University Press.

Pérez Medina, Tomás. 1998. *La Santería Cubana: El camino de Osha. Ceremonias, ritos, y secretos.* Madrid: Biblioteca Nueva.

Pérez Sarduy, Pedro, and Jean Stubbs. 1993. Introduction: The Rite of Social Communication. In *Afrocuba: An Anthology of Cuban Writing on Race, Politics and Culture*, edited by Pedro Pérez Sarduy and Jean Stubbs. London: Latin America Bureau.

―――. 2000. Introduction: Race and the Politics of Memory in Contemporary Black Cuban Consciousness. In *Afro-Cuban Voices: On Race and Identity in Contemporary Cuba*, edited by Pedro Pérez Sarduy and Jean Stubbs. Gainesville: University Press of Florida.

Rabkin, Rhoda P. 1991. *Cuban Politics: The Revolutionary Experiment*. New York: Praeger.

Ramos, Miguel. 1996. Afro-Cuban Orisha Worship. In *Santería Aesthetics in Contemporary Latin American Art*, edited by Arturo Lindsay. Washington, D.C.: Smithsonian Institution Press.

Rappaport, Roy A. 1979. *Ecology, Meaning, and Religion*. Berkeley, Calif.: North Atlantic Books.

Rodríguez Reyes, Andrés. 2000. Aro: La enfermedad y la regla de ocha. *Del Caribe* 32:72–77.

Roig y Mesa, Juan T. 1988 [1945]. *Plantas medicinales, aromáticas o venenosas de Cuba*. Havana: Editorial Cientifico-Tecnica.

Rosendahl, Mona. 1997a. *Inside the Revolution: Everyday Life in Socialist Cuba*. Ithaca, N.Y.: Cornell University Press.

―――. 1997b. The Ever-Changing Revolution. In *The Current Situation in Cuba: Challenges and Alternatives*, edited by Mona Rosendahl. Stockholm: Institute of Latin American Studies.

Sandoval, Mercedes C. 1975. *La religion afrocubana*. Madrid: Playor.

―――. 1977. Santeria: Afrocuban Concepts of Disease and Its Treatment in Miami. *Journal of Operational Psychiatry* 8(2):52–63.

―――. 1979. Santeria as a Mental Health Care System: A Historical Overview. *Social Science and Medicine* 13B (April):137–51.

―――. 1982. Thunder over Miami: Changó in a Technological Society. In *Thunder over Miami: Ritual Objects and AfroCuban Religion*, program notes for exhibition at University Gallery, University of Florida, September 7–October 17. Center for African Studies, University of Florida.

―――. 1995. Afro-Cuban Religion in Perspective. In *Enigmatic Powers: Syncretism with African and Indigenous Peoples' Religions among Latinos*, edited by Anthony M. Stevens-Arroyo and Andres I. Pérez y Mena. New York: Bildner Center for Western Hemisphere Studies.

Scheper-Hughes, Nancy. 1992. *Death without Weeping: The Violence of Everyday Life in Brazil*. Berkeley: University of California Press.

Scott, Rebecca. J. 1985. *Slave Emancipation in Cuba: The Transition to Free Labor, 1860–1899*. Princeton, N.J.: Princeton University Press.

Segal, Ronald. 1995. *The Black Diaspora*. London: Faber and Faber.

Seoane Gallo, Jose. 1988. *El folclor médico de Cuba*. Havana: Editorial de Ciencias Sociales.

Sjørslev, Inger. 2001. Possession and Syncretism: Spirits as Mediators in Modernity. In *Reinventing Religions: Syncretism and Transformation in Africa and the Americas*, edited by Sidney M. Greenfield and André Droogers. Lanham, Md.: Rowman and Littlefield Publishers.

Stoller, Paul, and Cheryl Olkes. 1987. *In Sorcery's Shadow: A Memoir of Apprenticeship among the Songhay of Niger*. Chicago: University of Chicago Press.

Strathern, Andrew, and Pamela J. Stewart. 1999. *Curing and Healing: Medical Anthropology in Global Perspective*. Durham, N.C.: Carolina Academic Press.

Stubbs, Jean. 1989. *Cuba: Test of Time*. London: Latin American Bureau.

Suchlicki, J. 2000. Castro's Cuba: Continuity instead of Change. In *Cuba: The Contours of Change*, edited by Susan K. Purcell and David J. Rothkopf. Boulder, Colo.: Lynne Rienner Publishers.

Thomas, Hugh. 1997. *The Slave Trade: The Story of the Atlantic Slave Trade: 1440–1870*. New York: Simon and Schuster.

Thompson, Robert F. 1983. *Flash of the Spirit: African and Afro-American Art and Philosophy*. New York: Random House.

Thylefors, Markel. 2002. Poverty and Sorcery in Urban Haiti. Ph.D. diss., Department of Social Anthropology, Göteborg University, Sweden.

Turner, Edith. 1992. *Experiencing Ritual: A New Interpretation of African Healing*. Philadelphia: University of Pennsylvania Press.

Turner, Victor W. 1967. *The Forest of Symbols: Aspects of Ndembu Ritual*. Ithaca, N.Y.: Cornell University Press.

———. 1969. *The Ritual Process: Structure and Anti-Structure*. Chicago: Aldine.

———. 1985. Body, Brain, and Culture. In *On the Edge of the Bush: Anthropology as Experience*, edited by Edith Turner. Tucson: University of Arizona Press.

———. 1986. Dewey, Dilthey, and Drama: An Essay in the Anthropology of Experience. In *The Anthropology of Experience*, edited by Victor W. Turner and Edward M. Bruner. Urbana: University of Illinois Press.

UNICEF. 2002. Official Summary. The State of the World's Children 2002: Leadership. http://www.unicef.org/sowc02summary/u5mranking.html (2003-01-22).

Valdés Garriz, Yrmino. 1997. *Dilogún*. Havana: Ediciones Unión.

Vélez, María T. 2000. *Drumming for the Gods: The Life and Times of Felipe García Villamil, Santero, Palero, Abakuá*. Philadelphia: Temple University Press.

Voeks, Robert A. 1997. *Sacred Leaves of Candomblé: African Magic, Medicine, and Religion in Brazil*. Austin: University of Texas Press.

Whyte, Susan R. 1997. *Questioning Misfortune: The Pragmatics of Uncertainty in Eastern Uganda*. Cambridge: Cambridge University Press.

Willis, Roy. 1999. *Some Spirits Heal, Others Only Dance: A Journey into Human Selfhood in an African Village*. Oxford: Berg.

Zimbalist, A. 2000. Whither the Cuban Economy? In *Cuba: The Contours of Change*, edited by Susan K. Purcell and David J. Rothkopf. Boulder, Colo.: Lynne Rienner Publishers.

Index

Page references in italics refer to illustrations

Letras (divination signs), 10, 48, 94–97, 177,
188; del año, 97–98
Lewis, Oscar, 4, 158
Lidia (santera), 122–23
Life switch. *See* Cambio de vida
Liminality, in initiations, 101, 140
Limpiezas (ritual cleansings), 50, 80, 98,
188; following divination, 93; in illness,
118; for mental stress, 137; for sorcery,
59–60
Liquids, hot and cool, 65
Lucia (santera), 152–56
Lucumí (ritual language), 188; in divination,
99; in possessions, 14; prayers in, 68. *See
also* Yorubas
Luis (babalao), 149–52; on exploitation, 159

Madrinas (godmothers), 104, 188; ritual
links to, 66
Magic: African, 52; slaves' use of, 55
Mal de ojo (evil eye), 189; because of envy,
58, 60; herbal remedies for, 77; protection
from, 135
Mandinga tribe, 185n3
Mano de Orula (ritual), 50, 105–6, 189
Manuals, santería, 38, 159
Maria (narrator), critique of santería, 160–61
Mariel boatlift, 143
Mario (santera), 145–48, 152
Marks, Morton, 77
Mastuerzo (plant), 78
Matanzas (Cuba): divination in, 92; iyabós
in, 104; poor neighborhoods of, 11, 36,
157; santería in, 8, 9
Matilda (santera), 7, 10–13, 27; initiation of,
11–12
Máximo (santero), 16–18, 26–27
Medicine: alternative, 177; chemical, 42, 45;
"green," 42, 45. *See also* Biomedicine,
Western
Medicine, herbal, xii, 4; administration of,
78; in medio asiento, 80; in palo monte,
42, 45; physicians' use of, 45, 121; in
santería, 42, 45, 74–80. *See also* Herbs;
Omiero
El Médico de la Salsa (singer), 58

Medio asiento (initiation), 20–21, 189; herbs
in, 80. *See also* Asiento
Menstrual blood: in palo monte, 54; in rituals, 65
Mercedes (santera), 138–40, 141
Metanlá (letra), 96, 123
Miami, santería in, 38
Misa espiritual (spiritual mass), 189; for illness, 26; possession in, 52
Montejo, Esteban, 30, 54, 55
Moyubbar (prayer), 68, 189
Muertos (spirits of dead), 189; aid from, 14;
as cause of illness, 47–48, 149; communi-
cation with, 88, 90; development of, 90;
in divination, 94; help from, 14; offerings
to, 18; possession by, 58, 60, 79; sorcery
involving, 134, 135–36; spiritist represen-
tation of, 53
Muertos oscuros (spirits), 48, 189; removal
of, 15
Murphy, Joseph M., 72
Music: Afro-Cuban, 174; in possession
trances, 71; in santería healing, 7, 109
Mythology, santería, 7, 123

Naciones (ethnic groups), 29
Narrators, 183–84
Native American healing, 52
Nature, santería view of, 113–15, 127
Necklaces. *See* Collares
Nervios (nerves), 22, 137, 189; biomedical
treatment of, 142–43; cofá de Orula for,
137; divination for, 137, 138, 140, 142; dur-
ing economic crisis, 40, 46; narratives
of, 136–43; rogación de cabeza for, 110;
santería treatment for, 51; social context
of, 142
New York, santería in, 38
Ngangas. *See* Prendas (cauldrons)
Nigeria: cultural exchanges with, 174; divi-
nation in, 92; initiation in, 116; religion
of, 2, 34, 177
Nyole, divination among, 93

Obara (letra), 95–96
Obatalá (divinity), 21, 189; attributes of, 82,
87; birthday of, 106; children of, 82, 87,

Santos: as aspect of nature, 113–15; attributes of, 89; as cause of illness, 50; children of, 87, 100, 104; collares of, 99; colors of, 89; communication from, 47, 64, 176; food for, 90; healing powers of, 87; minor, 86–87; offerings to, 64, 68, 69; palo monte equivalents of, 54; protection by, 131; punishment by, 48, 49–50, 87, 89, 118; reception of, 98–99; Yoruba names of, 30. *See also* Orishas

Sasafrás (plant), 78

Self: in anthropology, 109; and body, 117; boundaries, 58; of initiates, 109–10, 176; interpenetration with others, 111; in possession trances, 110; relation with objects, 111; in santería healing, 5, 8, 109–10, 112–13, 115, 133, 148, 156, 177; in Yoruba belief, 115

Sexual activity, abstinence from, 51, 101

Shangó (divinity), 190; altars of, 17, 68; attributes of, 84; birthday of, 106; color of, 107; communications from, 150; in dance, 71; as hot divinity, 65; initiates of, 11, 87, 100, 147; myths of, 57, 84, 88, 123; objects of, 67, 73; plants of, 77; popularity of, 84; possession by, 50, 107; punishment by, 88; as ruler of year, 98; sacrifices to, 112; as Siete Rayos, 54

Shaponna (divinity), 85

Silvia (santera), 145–48, 152

Slavery, abolition of, 31

Slaves: Congolese, 53–54; creation of culture, 185n2; tribal groups, 185n3; use of magic, 55

Slaves, Yoruba, 115; religious beliefs of, 2

Slave trade, 2, 27; banning of, 28

Social relations: in biomedicine, 119; role in illness, xiii, 2, 6, 27, 47, 110, 116, 121, 122, 127, 132, 135, 177; in santería, 8, 93, 110, 111, 148; in santería healing, 127, 148, 152; and sorcery, 111

Soperas (tureens), 67, 190; in initiations, 100

Sorcery, 53–62; agents of, 57; bodily fluids

in, 57; causes of, 56–57; cleansing for, 59–60; cures for, 111; discourse of, 63; divination concerning, 24, 56–58, 93, 95, 96, 130; during economic crisis, 56; and egoism, 60, 62; and espiritismo, 130; existential dimension of, 63–64; herbal protection against, 78, 79; illness through, xiii, 48, 49, 56, 58–59, 62–64, 109, 121; involving muertos, 134, 135–36; narratives of, 128–36; in palo monte, 14, 48, 132; physicians' belief in, 119; protection from, 14, 64, 130; rituals combating, 132; rumors of, 58; skepticism concerning, 15; and social relations, 111; *versus* witchcraft, 185n1. *See also* Palo monte

Spirits: development of, 53; removal of, 59–60. *See also* Muertos (spirits of dead)

Spiritual baths, 8; following consultations, 49; for nervios, 51, 137; plants in, 77

Star-shake (plant), 55

Sticks, in palo monte, 54

Stress, mental. *See* Illness, mental; Nervios

Tableros (divining trays), 21, 92

Ta José (spirit), 168

Tambores (drum ceremonies), 12, 70, 155, 190; *para egún*, 106. *See also* Bembés; Drums, ritual

Teresa (Pentecostal), 163–64, 166–67, 170, 171

Torricelli-Graham Act (1996), 41

Tourism, Cuban, 15, 35, 36; Afro-Cuban culture in, 174; Afro-Cuban religions in, 171; for health, 39

Trabajo (spiritual work), 190

Trinidad, Yoruba in, 30

Turner, Edith, 72

Turner, Victor W., 101

United States, santería in, xi, 38

Los Van Van (salsa group), 16

Violín para Oshún (ritual), 106

Virgen de la Candelaria, 85

Virgen de la Caridad del Cobre, 84, 90

Johan Wedel is an instructor in social
anthropology at Göteborg University, Sweden.